THE *BEST* POSSIBLE YOU

THE *BEST* POSSIBLE YOU

*A unique nutritional guide
to healing your body*

HANNAH RICHARDS

S

First published in Great Britain in 2020 by Orion Spring
This paperback edition published in 2020 by Orion Spring
an imprint of The Orion Publishing Group Ltd
Carmelite House, 50 Victoria Embankment
London EC4Y 0DZ

An Hachette UK Company

1 3 5 7 9 10 8 6 4 2

A CIP catalogue record for this book is
available from the British Library.

ISBN (mass market paperback) 978 1 4091 6471 5

Typeset by Input Data Services Ltd, Somerset

Printed and bound in Great Britain by Clays Ltd, Elcograf S.p.A.

www.orionbooks.co.uk

To my sister, Clare – my love love

HEALTH ADVICE AND CAUTION

CONTENTS

INTRODUCTION

Imagine if you possessed the knowledge to read your body and also listen to it so you could make the right decisions for your own health. It would certainly save you time and money – visits to the doctor and numerous prescriptions – and that, I suppose, is the main reason why I wrote this book.

Your body tells you what is going on, you just have to listen to it. The world of health is everywhere, and sometimes it feels like it cannot be escaped. Every shop window and every magazine cover sings the virtues of being healthy. There is always a new supplement on the market, there is always a new superfruit in town, there is always a new advertising campaign 'shaming' people into thinness. But what is health and what does healthy mean? Are you healthy because you do not have a regular prescription or haven't been to the doctor's in a year or three? Are you healthy because you're a size 0? Is being healthy a competition, is it about being vain? Is it something to feel smug about or is it something to be ashamed of, because so many people are sick and overweight?

The aim of this book is to teach you how you can improve and better your own health by getting back to basics. To learn and under-stand where food comes from. To get back in touch with your body and build a relationship with every part, every organ and system that it houses. This book will help you heal yourself when you're sick or run-down or have a problem you need to solve, but it will also help you to keep every bit of your body well maintained so you can be the best possible you. I wrote this book to teach you the fundamentals of how the body works, what the body is capable of doing and, crucially, what you can do to ensure that you are the best possible version of you. The human body is often unquestioned, if it works; it is only when it starts to malfunction that we say, 'I'd better start looking after myself.' But prevention is so much better than the cure, and when the body is not sick it is so simple to look after it and understand it.

As a nutritional therapist and lifestyle coach, I find most of my clients come to me because their regular doctor, using mainstream medicine, hasn't been able to find a cause for the tiredness or bloating or headaches they are experiencing, or because the drugs they (usually) have been given to treat these maladies – antidepressants, anti-inflammatories or iron pills – haven't helped.

I believe that this suggests there is a gap in the way in which medicine works at the moment. The treatments your doctor can offer are designed to deal with just one thing, such as heartburn or not being able to sleep, but they won't be able to deal with your system as a whole. Your doctor is trained to tell you what is medically wrong with you and prescribe something to treat it, but it doesn't always get to the root of the problem, physically or emotionally, and therefore ensure that it will not recur.

My approach is different, I am not that interested in looking for what's most obviously wrong right now, but in the bigger picture, the long term – where you are and have been on the paradigm of health. Once we know this, together we can decide on preventative measures for the future, rather than sending you away with a one-off prescription only for you to come back six months later to receive the same diagnosis yet again, or something else as a result of not tackling the root of the issue properly.

This approach, known as functional or integrated medicine, makes a lot of sense to me and is one that I'm happy to say seems to be interesting a growing number of doctors, too. It aims to make full use of conventional medicine – antibiotics and emergency surgery are most certainly life-savers – but in addition it recognises the importance of the relationship between the practitioner and the client, and how nutrition and lifestyle changes can get your whole system working in a healthier, more efficient way.

This book gives a breakdown of the important organs that are inside you, what their jobs entail, when and how it can go wrong and how to heal it back to health. We have four 'bodies' in this human body of ours – the spiritual, emotional, nutritional and physical – and a healthy body relies on all these elements to be in tune with each other for the absence of disease. If you only look after one body you will find malfunction or a state of disease creeps in somewhere else. There is no hierarchy to the body; it requires a plethora of complex systems and pathways to work together like a beautiful dance. Only then will you experience the vast abilities of the body you live in and what it is capable of! Sounds easy? It is. You've just lost your mojo and I'm going to show you how to get it back.

The trouble with how we eat today

Nutrition is the most written-about subject of our time – you only have to look around you to see how many different recipe books are being produced with a healthy eating slant. I love cookbooks, but not everyone is best equipped to write them. I want to read recipes written by someone who has eaten that dish, tried it time and time again, who has experimented with foods and flavours and is able to bring to you the wisdom, love and knowledge of their passion for food and nutrition. It's that information that I'm aiming to bring you with this book.

What we need to remember is that there is no one food that is going to save you from disease, make you thinner, clear up your spots, make you taller or more intelligent. If you continue to search for the perfect diet you'll only create anxiety, and that's one of the biggest health problems we have in the developed world at the moment; anxiety over what to eat, when to eat, how to eat, with whom to eat, etc. You cannot turn a corner, swipe right or open a magazine without being blatantly told that what you are eating is wrong – but I say ignore all this, listen to your body and go with what makes you feel well. In this book I'll share with you nutritional and lifestyle plans that will help you.

It is not surprising that no one knows how to eat when all the people who have a voice are destroying the relationship we have with food. Health bloggers and vegan advocates have just swapped one addiction of overeating for another of neurotic eating, they just don't know it, and TV documentaries often miss the opportunity to educate the public about healthy eating. We shame the fat, we praise the thin, but ultimately neither group is getting the information they need. We need a different approach, we need to get back to embracing our bodies and the natural way in which they work.

Sadly, we are also seeing the demise of independent fishmongers, greengrocers, butchers and bakers. These expert food sellers know the provenance of their products and are selling quality, locally pro-duced ingredients. Often these shops have been there for generations but are now at risk of extinction, and that's a real shame, because with them goes their expertise.

This loss of connection to our foods is troubling because eating seasonal foods native to our countries is important for all aspects of our health, and that of the planet. In the 1930s, dentist Weston A. Price travelled to meet with Australian Aborigines, New Zealand Maoris, African tribes and the residents of remote villages in Switzerland to study the health of populations untouched by Western civilisa-tion. He wanted to discover the factors behind good dental health, and during his travels he discovered that deformed dental arches, overcrowded teeth and cavities were all the result of nutritional de-ficiencies and not inherited genetic defects, as had been previously thought. The people in the groups he observed all had good straight teeth, free from decay; they had strong physiques, good disease resis-tance. He concluded that this was a result of their nutritionally rich diet, consuming foods native to their lands. And this is the crucial part – there wasn't a denatured, refined, processed, canned, heated, treated, bleached, packaged, hydrogenated, low-fat, toxic, artificial, powdered, coloured or blue food product to be found.

Instead all these groups of traditional cultures consumed animal protein, fat from fish, water and land fowl, eggs, milk and milk products, insects and reptiles. They ate what was available to them and their diets were far higher in calcium and other minerals, fats, etc. than the average Western diet. This primitive diet is also naturally high in enzymes, and Price didn't find anyone suffering from IBS. The food was raw, fermented and naturally preserved; nuts and grains were soaked, and fruit, vegetables and meats were all eaten in season.

This simplistic way of eating is what we need to strive to return to. As the race to take control of our food becomes ever more poignant, Michael Pollan's book *Food Rules* becomes the food bible of the twenty-first century.[1] One of my favourite rules of his is 'eat like your grandmother did'. I say to my clients, if it has a pair of eyes, a tail, a pair of wings or four legs you can eat it. If it fell from a tree or grew from the ground then you can have it, safe in the knowledge that it is from the earth and natural. However, if it did none of those things, or the main ingredient of your dish did none of those things, question how it came to take up residence in your fridge or on your plate. For example, if the label says 'low-fat' or 'fat-free', it probably means 'high-sugar' and 'high-carbohydrate', because fat is the macronutrient that makes you feel satisfied and adds flavour and depth to food; if the fats have been taken out you can be sure that sugar and chemicals have been added in. Labels also shouldn't have to tell you things that you can see, for example, 'natural'. This is what our eyes are for.

Obesity

Integrated medicine, which I practise, involves a wide-angled view of health, looking at the way we move as well as the way we eat. This approach acknowledges what an amazing and resilient system the human body is; our bodies are a legacy from generations of humans who survived times of astonishing hardship – plagues, famine, extremes of heat and cold. It is ironic that today our bodies are being threatened by the world of plenty and comfort that our technologies have created. This new twenty-first-century lifestyle is challenging our bodies in ways that they have never faced before. How can we expect our bodies to thrive as they once did when exercise now involves little more than sitting at home playing video games, and hunting has been replaced with a drive to the supermarket to pick up a snack packed with sugar and other refined carbohydrates?

It may come as no surprise that the greatest causes of obesity in children and adolescents today are video games and TV. Today, obesity is at its peak the world over, having more than doubled since 1980, and child obesity in particular is soaring.[2] In 2017 the Organisation for Economic Co-operation and Development (OECD) stated that more than 50 per cent of adults and one in six children are overweight or obese within the countries they surveyed (of which there are 34 in the OECD[3]), observing that the rates were highest in the US, Mexico, New Zealand and Hungary (the lowest were in Japan and Korea).[4] Furthermore, the World Health Organization found that throughout the world, 41 million children under the age of five were estimated to be overweight in 2016, with the majority living in Asia and a quarter living in Africa. A startling reality is that most of the world's population[5] live in countries where obesity kills more people than being underweight does. Yet the most staggering point to be made here – and probably the most obvious – is that obesity is preventable.

Today we find that even in developed countries there is a sea of malnourishment; this is surprising because we tend to think it is a problem that only developing or war-torn nations have to deal with. In fact, most overweight people are malnourished because they are devoid of nutrients, vitamins and minerals, which is due to the over-processed and over-refined foods that are on offer in abundance, which keep us all firmly addicted and co-dependent on these drug-like foods. The best thing we can do for our health is to eat a varied, nutritious diet – one that is full of colourful fruits and vegetables, fish, meats, nuts and seeds – whose provenance we know and which are, preferably, produced organically and seasonally.

Despite the fact that we have more knowledge about healthy lifestyles than previous generations, we are all now fatter and sicker. For those who want to lose weight, there is always a new diet or theory on how to be leaner, how to eat cleaner, but these only work for a while. Many of these diets don't teach you about you, about how you feel about food, about what you crave, when you crave it and why you crave it. Part of the problem is not being present when eating our food; many of us concentrate more on our phones or our screens than what's on our plates and this leads to a disconnect, which is where problems with digestion start. The phone has become such an extension of our being that separating ourselves from it creates anxiety, which does not bode well for optimal digestion. However, reassuringly, this is a problem that can quite easily be solved and can help you on the road to good health.

I believe that weight loss is easy; you simply have to figure out what caused you to become overweight in the first place, then this becomes the start of the story. Understand this, and you are on your way to better health. People who avoid doing this, who simply look for a quick fix by counting their calories, go for low-fat options and watch what they eat, spend an inordinate amount of time being unhappy. I watch them leave my clinic as fat as they arrived; they come to me looking for a speedy solution because the plethora of diets they have tried have not worked. People who are addicted to dieting or who are in search of the body beautiful are like serial divorcees; they keep making the same mistake. They don't want to delve into that area of untapped potential and unravel the emotion, pain, hurt and angst that being overweight or neurosis covers up, so instead they continue to take the same journey until they decide enough is enough.

Counting calories, typing out what you have eaten and putting it into a spreadsheet is a full-time job. I get stressed out looking at the charts and plans and macronutrients that some clients bring in. I barely look at them, to be honest, because it is not how life should be lived – there is another way!

The straw that broke the camel's back

In addition to poor diet and inactive lifestyles, another contributory factor to the rising levels of obesity is that we are now being exposed to a massive rise in electromagnetic energies and more chemicals than at any time in history. All this has a powerful impact on our metabolic system, which might be described as the way we use food and energy. So it's not surprising that we are facing an epidemic of metabolic diseases such as diabetes, obesity, cancer and depression.

Sounds gloomy and depressing? Don't worry, here's the good news: you can change the direction you are going in. Integrated functional medicine enables you to put yourself in the driving seat with regard to your health so that you can make choices that make you feel energetic and positive. The lifestyle changes you can make can be incredibly simple: such as drinking more water, taking a walk every day, seeing something new each day, writing down your thoughts or meeting up with friends. However, when these changes are new to you, they can be hard to stick to on a regular basis. This is why once I've identified the changes that need to be made I work with my clients every step of the way, ensuring that the changes are easy, doable, practical and necessary. And this is what I'm going to help you on your way towards in this book.

There is so much more to this than the simplistic formula for healthy living that you may sometimes hear from doctors: 'It all comes down to moving a bit more and eating a bit less.' That sounds sensible – after all, if you don't burn your calories they will be stored as fat. Yet the wonderful American science journalist Gary Taubes, who was the first person to explain why saturated fat wasn't a heart attack on a plate, believes the idea that calories in should equal calories out 'has done more damage to the health world than any other single statement'. What makes it so appealing, he says, is that it makes 'Obesity the penalty for gluttony and sloth'[6]. This has been enshrined as commonsense wisdom for 50-plus years and it's time to take it down.

The best way by which we can take control of our health is to be more aware of the food we eat, the way we move, the thoughts we think and the hours we sleep. What you eat makes you who you are, what you absorb makes you able to be who you are, and how you eliminate waste products from the body allows you to be the best that you can be.

In the UK and the USA, statistics show that a poor diet is the main contributor to early death and chronic onset disease. Second on the list after diet for causing the most deaths is high blood pressure, followed by the importance of children's and their mothers' nutrition. So hopefully this highlights the magnitude of the role that food plays in our life as regards staying healthy or getting sick. (If you want to know, smoking is actually fourth on the list.[7] You might be surprised at this; many still believe that smoking is the primary cause of death the world over. In a way it is good that so many people still believe this; if you were around in the 1950s you would be mistaken for assuming that smoking would further your life expectancy, digestion, lifestyle and social status, and this misinformation came from the demi-gods in white coats. Doctors in the 1950s were set on a pedestal, and if they said it or did it then their patients followed suit. My favourite smoking campaigns in the 1950s were 'More doctors smoke Camels than any other cigarette'[8], and this second ad produced in 1969, 'Blow in her face and she'll follow you anywhere'.)

Many diseases are preventable through good nutrition; those we have had for centuries, such as gout (which implies we have always had a struggle with food), type 2 diabetes, insulin resistance, obesity, high blood sugar, cancer and auto-immune diseases. So why isn't healthy eating the first piece of advice that comes out of doctors' surgeries the world over? Giving advice on food empowers and educates the client and takes the burden off the healthcare system, as food has the power to heal. However, this is not happening on a big enough scale the world over.

There are a few simple prerequisites to being a highly efficient, all-cylinders-firing, functional human being:

1. Optimum and intelligent food sourcing and selection.
2. Optimum digestion and absorption and elimination.
3. Optimum hydration levels.
4. Optimum sleep.
5. Optimum movement – tuning in and tuning out.

Failing to meet these needs is the top reason why people find their way to me, but these five things are all you need to help yourself on the way to the best possible you. My philosophy is that if you look after your physiology by looking after your cells, you won't have to 'fix' a pathology. And if you look after your cells, they will look after your blood, your immune system, organs, body and health.

So, put simply, your cells should be number one on your list of priorities. Why are our cells so important? That's all your body really is – just a whole bunch of cells getting together and forming larger structures. They are like the worker bees toiling under the queen bee – you!

When a cell divides it passes on a DNA legacy – a blueprint to tell the next cell how to work. All cells are the same in classical composition and require energy and ATP (adenosine triphosphate). They also have memories, and their ability to remember all your past experiences with influence is communicated in the cells of the body all the time.

We can't talk about cells without talking about mitochondria. All cells contain mitochondria, and it is these mitochondria that allow oxygen to be transported around the body via the red blood cells.

Welcome to the powerhouse that converts energy from the food we eat into energy for the hundreds of biological reactions and processes that need to take place. So when you consider that the mitochondria in the cells are essential for energy production and the cells are the building blocks for every tissue, organ, ligament and tendon in the body, it seems obvious that looking after your cells should be your priority for optimum health.

What is good nutrition?

Nutrition should not be complicated, which is why at the heart of my advice there are a few simple tips: keep it simple, eat organic, eat seasonal and make your meals from scratch with your own hands. Nourishing your body needs to be a high priority, so start reevaluating what is important and focus on these things to create a life that you want, because if you do, you can have everything you dream of! Don't see eating well as cutting out what you love; it's about supporting your current lifestyle with appropriate measures to improve your current state of health, either physically, chemically or emotionally.

Good nutrition starts in the soil. We are humans; we are living organisms that have originated from the soil, the earth. The problem is, soil is not what it used to be and its integrity has been jeopardised by the use of chemicals and fertilisers that have been added to it to grow crops bigger and faster to produce more for our expanding population. As a result, the soil has a decreased nutritional value, and this affects the whole food chain; the plants are eaten not only by us but also by the animals which we in turn eat, so ultimately we all get sicker because the nutritional levels in these foods have been depleted. Food is not what it used to be. Do not be fooled by a big, beefy red tomato or a perfectly shaped apple. Vegetables are at their most beautiful when they are ugly – then they have character, as they have struggled to get to the top of the land – so try looking for fruit and vegetables that still have a bit of mud on them or ones that are not perfectly formed or aesthetically pleasing to the eye. The only packaging your food should be covered in is mud and you'll find these products at a farmers' market, farm shop or grown at home. These products also increase your gut microbiome, so it's like a two-for-one deal at the supermarket, except this one is way better! The more remnants from the land your food has, the fewer refining processes it will have been through before it got onto your plate, so the more likely it is that it has a greater nutritional value and will be easier to digest.

This is basically where my beliefs come from, and what I am hoping to convey in this book. I am all about making what doesn't work, work better. That doesn't mean everyone needs to stop what they are doing, buy a blender and start blending their fridge into mush! It is about a journey, your journey, and not comparing anything you do with anyone else's lifestyle. You are as unique as your fingerprint, and what works for Nick next door or Sally at work will not always work for you. You need to learn how your body works, figure out what you want and then make some realistic plans to allow that dream to happen.

The human body is designed so carefully that it can and does heal itself, if only you will let it.

HOW THIS BOOK WORKS

Together we are going to go on a journey around the body, looking at all the areas that make up our wondrous anatomy and how we can best serve each of them so they will optimally serve us. You will find information, advice and 'actions' to perform to help you with this, as well as information on specific pathologies that might crop up with the organ in question and ways to prevent/treat them by looking at your nutrition, your movement and your emotions.

The energies and emotions of the body

As I've mentioned above, in this book we'll be looking at the spiritual, physical, emotional and nutritional sides of each organ as well as the scientific side. By looking after all these bodies you stand yourself in far better stead of being free from disease and enjoying everything that life has to offer.

As part of this, I will explain where the meridians of the organ in question lie.[9] The meridian describes the overall energy distribution style of Chinese medicine and gives us a basic understanding of how Qi, energy, blood and fluids permeate the entire body. A meridian is a road of energy that flows from one point to another, a line you can't see but can sense and feel. The meridians take up residency in a similar way to the plethora of branching veins and arteries in the circulatory system and can be mapped – they have parallel lines running together, with each meridian having acupuncture points along the way. Unlike the circulatory system, the physiology and anatomy of the meridians is not fixed and the meridians have more of an energetic manifestation that flows and stagnates depending on the health and vitality of the body. Each organ has a meridian known as channels or vessels.

Case studies

You will also find real-life case studies about clients I have worked with to illustrate some of the pathologies mentioned. These people have gone on to change their physiology through many of the nutrition and lifestyle recommendations in this book. This should help you to visualise how you too can prevent and reverse disease by getting back to the basics.

Nutrition plan

You will find a sample meal plan for each organ with all the foods that can benefit and heal it. You don't necessarily need to follow the whole day every day, but sample one of the meals. This section contains general health advice and can be followed by anyone wanting to improve their nutritional and lifestyle habits.

Pathologies

The chapter then looks at some common pathologies or problems that can occur with the organ and shows you how you might look at the healing process through a different set of eyes.

Top tips

Make sure to read over the 10 top tips at the end of each chapter, which will help you keep your health a priority. They are easy and doable and will help you to be the best possible you.

STOP MAKING EATING FROM SCRATCH DIFFICULT – JUST DO IT

Here is my tried-and-tested tipping-point plan, which you can easily incorporate into your life. When the wine flows more than water, the gym calls you more than your mother and a muffin top takes up residence on your belt (just some of the reasons why you might need a helping hand to make changes – see the list below), you need this plan to get it together! If you embark on one of the popular weight-loss plans you will, inevitably, fail at some point. Similarly, if you embark on a fitness plan you will also fail at some point, because neither is sustainable in the long run. Successfully becoming healthier is about mindset; at the heart of looking after yourself is being kind to yourself and loving yourself, and a plan that is doomed to fail will not help this. Getting in the right frame of mind will help you pull back when you need to and allow you to always see success and feel positive, as well as give you the tools to be the best possible you. There is no right or wrong; it is only important that you create the best nutrition and lifestyle plan that will achieve optimum wellbeing, and this is what I am striving to do with this book, to make you the best possible you.

There are several ways of checking where you are on the optimal health scale, which will help you decide where you need to get to.

These include:

Blood pressure: This is recorded with two numbers; the systolic pressure (higher number) is the force at which your heart pumps blood around your body, and the diastolic pressure (lower number) is the resistance to the blood flow in the blood vessels. They're both measured in millimetres of mercury (mmHg). Ideally you want a reading of 120/80, which means that your blood is flowing easily and happily through your blood vessels. So if you feel your blood boiling or your capillaries flooding your cheeks (on a machine it may look like 140/90), this is your tipping point.

Happy weight: We all have a happy weight; a photo we want to aim to get back to, or a pair of trousers that give instant satisfaction when we wear them. So what's your happy weight? Whatever it is, think back to how you felt and what you did to get there. Then recognise what you did after that point to fall out of the happy weight zone. So have a cold shower or give yourself a slight slap around the face or a good old talking to in the mirror and sort yourself out with an intention to get back on the straight and narrow. As a guideline, if your waist is over 80cm (31½ inches) for women and 94cm (37 inches) for men it's time for positive change!

Blood glucose: Another great marker of health. Remember that even if you are skinny or lean that does not mean you are exempt from having high levels of sugar in the blood. So when eating a whole packet of sweets seems normal or the glass of wine once a week is now 2–3 glasses every night, and you find you are craving sugar after every meal, you may well be at tipping point.

Your blood glucose levels should be on waking (fasting) under 100 mg/dl, then between 70 and 99 mg/dl before meals and under 140 mg/dl at two hours after meals. You can check these levels with your local surgery by asking for a HbA1c test.

Body fat: You can measure this with calipers or use an electronic scale. If you pick up your skin and measure with calipers you want a few things to happen: you should be able to pick the fat up and roll the fat off the muscle. These are both signs of healthy body tissue and that you have a good diet. Ideally you need to be able to separate the muscle from the fat tissue and only measure the fat tissue. Body fat levels for men should be 15–20 per cent, and for women should be 24–30 per cent. You can measure from 7–19 different sites on the body to work out the overall body fat percentage.

Urine: There is a simple and easy test that I use with all clients at the Gut Clinic, which uses their urine to check their pH levels, glucose, protein, yeast, blood and much more. It is simple to do yourself, though (you can buy home kits online).

Sleep: If more often than not you get into bed after midnight and you are feeling fat, fed up and fatigued, then the first thing to do is to get into bed earlier! Let's keep it simple; your body repairs itself when you go to bed; it needs to rest from the emotional, physical and chemical stress you throw at it every day. So many people say to me they sleep 12 hours and are really good sleepers; my response is that, if so, you don't have the fuel to wake up and people who sleep 12 hours do not wake up refreshed. They wake up and if they don't fall straight back to sleep they struggle until they reach for a mug and the beautiful black stuff passes their lips! Do not be fooled by people who sleep for nearly half of the day.

As well as the above factors, you will know if it's time to make a change if you don't do the following things:

Do you?

- Drink at least 2 litres (3½ pints) of clear filtered water every day?
- Eat without your phone or away from your computer?

- Move your body in a different range of speeds and directions each day?
- Break into a sweat and get out of breath?
- Spend time being still?
- Spend time outside?
- Eat food that is green and has come from the soil?
- Smile and laugh and speak to other people regularly?
- See, do or go somewhere new every day?

These are the things you need to be aiming for, which, along with the nutritional advice I've packed this book with, are going to help you get to the best possible you. We all know that such changes take time, and time has become the richest commodity that we trade, so work through these carefully and at your own pace, following the guidelines below.

Set a daily intention: Sometimes setting too many goals can be more stressful than it is beneficial, so instead set just one daily intention; that way you are more likely to follow through. Think, what is the one thing you need to do today? What will make you feel calmer and more in control of your life? It might be to pick up the dry cleaning that's been in the shop for four weeks, or it could be not to raise your voice in the office. By having an intention you are more likely to design a plan that you succeed at rather than fail at.

Photos: Take these at the start; front, side and back and then again every four weeks to assess your progress, to see what that beautiful body of yours looks like, to help you to get comfortable with looking at it and embracing every part of it. Taking measurements for your weight and around your waist, hips and inner thighs are all a starting point but it's about how you feel. If you can associate how you feel with how you look you can start to create a more healthy mental relationship with your body, rather than chasing the numbers on the scale.

Movement: Your body is designed to move, so if you only move in gear 1, i.e. you walk everywhere slowly and never break sweat, you probably need to explore what gear 4 or even 5 looks like and give your visceral body a good old workout! Movement does not have to look like a gym membership or being part of a running group, it can simply be a 10-minute bodyweight workout in your garden or living room. It can be riding your bike, dancing or making love to your partner. The point is, the body must move and the body must sweat.

Do therapy: We often think that therapy is only for 'real issues' – 'traumas'. It is a very British thing to keep our thoughts and feelings to ourselves, in the hope that they will magically go away. Well, this is not a theory I subscribe to. Identifying the issues and being aware of the issues is a good starting point. Writing things down is another good starting point and perhaps easier, too, as you can tear the page out and no one gets to see what you've written, but what you have done by talking or writing is to release the thought, issue or problem that is plaguing you. We commonly accept that the gym is the place for our physical body and the kitchen is the place for the nutritional body, so why not the therapist's chair or your notepad for your mental/emotional body?

Take a walk without your phone: Human beings spend so much time in offices with air conditioning, tied to our desks and a plethora of communication gadgets, which, among other things, depletes our microbiome as the environment is sterile. A walk outside challenges all bodies – the physical with the movement, the mental with taking in new surroundings, the emotional from the detachment from communication phobia, and at the same time increases the gut microbiome.

Love: Above all else, the giving and receiving of love makes the world go around. A gesture of kindness can make the difference between your day being mediocre or exceptional. The greatest love is you, though, and if you look after you, you can look after everyone else. If you are not your first priority in life you are putting someone else first and, by doing that, you create a pressure. The only person who should be sitting on a pedestal is you and your beautiful body.

Don't forget that you are in charge of your life, no one else. If something is not working, make the necessary change. That's what I am aiming to do in this book and in my daily work: to educate people to be their own doctor. Start by listening to your body and asking yourself what is not working as well as it used to. One thing is for sure, the more you listen, the more you will learn and the more your body will tell or show you, enabling you to optimise your body's health.

I believe that diet and nutrition should be at the forefront of every education system – there should be a programme and systems that incorporate therapeutic, alternative and preventative wellness programmes along with lifestyle changes, to promote a state of health and an enthusiasm for health. More importantly, all this should be put in place in order for the human body to be resilient to the pressures and toxins of the twenty-first-century healthcare model. This is what I hope to share with you in this book – an alternative way to the traditional medicinal approach to live well. So let's get started.

Footnotes

(1) Pollan, M., *Food Rules: An Eater's Manual* 6th Edn (New York, 2009).

(2) Obesity update 2017, www.oecd.org/health/obesity-update.htm (accessed on 03/05/2017).

(3) OECD Watch, www.oecdwatch.org/oecd-guidelines/oecd (accessed on 03/05/2017).

(4) Childhood, Overweight and Obesity, http://www.who.int/diet-physicalactivity/childhood/en/ (accessed on 21/08/16).

(5) Current World Population, http://www.worldometers.info/world-population/ (accessed on 11/01/2016).

(6) Taubes, G., *Why We Get Fat: And What to Do About It* (New York, 2010).

(7) Haidong Wang, Laura Dwyer-Lindgren, 'Age-specific and sex-specific mortality in 187 countries, 1970–2010: a systematic analysis for the Global Burden of Disease Study 2010', *The Lancet* (15 December 2012).

(8) 'More doctors smoke Camels than any other cigarette', this and other cigarette advertisements appeared in the American Medical Association's official journal, 1930s–50s.

(9) The information regarding the properties of each meridian (pp 61; 100; 130; 157; 196, 222; 245; 278) has been adapted primarily from Ted Andrews, *The Healer's Manual: A Beginner's Guide to Energy Healing for yourself and Others* (US, 2002).

1. THE SKIN

The Body's Boundary

Perhaps the most fascinating organ of the body, the skin is the body's boundary, on average stretching to cover a total area of 6 metres (20 feet). It is a boundary between the internal and external world, and its function, among other things, is to protect and serve the best possible you. The skin is often not seen as an organ at all, but it is in fact the largest organ. We all have different skin depending on our cultural make-up, heritage and genes. The skin you live in is as complex and clever as an encyclopedia, so let's make sure you're equipped to read and understand what it is telling you.

It is said that the eyes are the windows to your soul, but I like to think of your skin as the story of your life. Every little blemish tells a tale, every scar stems from a story. It's like looking into a crystal ball of your past, present and future health. During the first consultation with any client, I'll do something called 'face mapping', where I look at the condition of and elasticity of the skin on the face. Your skin is your curriculum vitae, your covering letter and book jacket all in one. Healthy skin reveals how old you are, how much you respect, feed and water your body. Face mapping gives you an immediate insight into the organs of the body and which ones could do with support, especially the liver, kidneys and the gastrointestinal tract (GIT), helping to build a symptom profile that enables us to put together a bespoke health plan. So, in our quest for the best possible you, the skin is a great place to start.

> The concept of face mapping is as old as man. Hippocrates, the shaman and traditional Chinese medicine all used it as a tool for diagnosis. It can show a weakness in the organ systems[1] and other systems of the body.
>
> - Spots around the chin line can indicate an hormonal imbalance.
> - Dark circles under the eyes can indicate the detoxification pathways need some support.
> - White or pale lips can indicate an iron deficiency.
> - Cracks at the corner of the mouth indicate low vitamin B2 levels.
>
> It is important to note that none of these signs alone are indicators of there being a disease state in an organ but rather are an indication that more investigation should happen. The signs simply suggest imbalances or inflammation in the organ system.

The body contains slightly more bacteria cells than human cells and we come into contact with numerous various potential pathogens (disease-causing microbes) every day, but the body does not get diseased every single day. This is because the skin is doing its job of protecting us. Think of the skin as a security company, with its main job being to provide safety in an unstable or insecure environment. Consider how robust your skin is, how many layers it has, how it stops you from bleeding to death or losing all the organs it houses. It is elastic and robust. It can regrow and heal itself – if you cut your skin it can (or should) heal pretty quickly.

It is a boundary, a fence that keeps everything in.

There are other structures in the body that share this security role, too, which work in conjunction with the skin; the brain is protected by the skull, and the heart and lungs by the ribs. The body is like an extended family, with every organ linked to another, ensuring everyone is happy and functioning to optimal levels.

In this chapter you will learn about the foods that help reduce inflammation in the body, ensuring beautiful-looking skin, as well as the best products to use (in order to avoid contact with harmful chemicals as much as possible). I will also share with you information and advice on some common skin conditions, how best to heal them and how to prevent them coming back.

Facts:

- Your skin covers on average 6 metres (20 feet) – the size of a boxing ring!
- Over 14 species of fungi live between your toes.
- Sweat is odourless; it's the bacteria that make the smell.
- When you are born, you don't get fingerprints until the third month.
- Your skin sheds 50,000 cells a minute.

A BIT MORE ANATOMY

There are three layers of the skin: the epidermis, the dermis and the hypodermis.

The **epidermis** is the outer layer, the skin you can touch; a tough, robust and protective layer which protects internal organs as well as muscles, nerves and blood vessels against trauma, such as an accident, car crash or fall. The cells in the epidermis are called keratinocytes and originate from the basal layer of the epidermis. These cells migrate slowly towards the surface of the skin and then shed, to be replaced by new cells. The average skin cell is replaced every 14–21 days.

Beneath the epidermis is the **dermis**, made mostly from collagen to create a thick layer of fibrous and elastic tissue. It is collagen that gives skin flexibility and strength. Within the dermis are nerve endings, sweat glands, sebaceous glands (small glands in the skin which secrete a lubricating oily matter (sebum) into the hair follicles to lubricate the skin and hair), hair follicles and blood vessels. The nerve endings sense feeling, pressure, pain, touch and temperature and are more sensitive in the extremities – the hands and feet. Think back to the last time you dropped something heavy onto your toe or shut your finger in the door – the pain can be off the Richter scale for a relatively small area, because of little things called somatosensory receptors whose job it is to sense pain.

Lastly, you have the fat layer, otherwise known as the **hypodermis**, which is the one we seem so concerned about removing! Its role is to insulate the body against hot and cold, and it serves as an energy storage system. Distribution of fat differs all over the body; the smallest layer covering the eyelid and the largest usually covering the abdomen or the buttocks. You will be aware of this layer on a cold day when the fatty parts of the body get cold, because there is less blood supply to these areas as they are not as metabolically active.

Did you know?

'In the buff' became synonymous for nude in seventeenth-century England. The term derives from soldiers' leather tunics, or 'buffs'. The light-brown colour of these apparently resembled a soldier's backside.

ENERGIES OF THE SKIN

The meridians of the skin

There are no meridians specifically for the skin, as the skin incorporates all the individual organ meridians. So when the skin shows a rash or a site of redness it will be as a result of the meridian of an organ passing through that area of the body. For example, red elbows may not be the problem of the skin but an imbalance in the lungs or the heart as the meridian lines pass through the elbows.

The emotions of the skin

Psychodermatology is the study of the psychological effects that the mind is having on the skin. Just as you cannot hide from your emotions, so you cannot hide from your skin – it is the biggest lie-detector you have! Like a colour chart, your face displays shades of anger, embarrassment, pain, shock, grief and confidence. It happens automatically and the physiological connection to the skin is inescapable. Any emotion can cause all your blood vessels to spontaneously open up so that your skin colour changes in seconds. It is for this reason that you can tell so much from your skin.

THE FOUR BODIES OF THE SKIN

The spiritual body

Your skin is the first thing you present to the world around you, and also reflects how you see yourself. Having healthy, glowing skin can often make us feel more confident about ourselves. When the skin is inflamed or blotchy we might want to hide away from the world, inwardly or outwardly. Any change in the skin reflects our moods and actions. It is easy just to think of the skin on our face but the skin is the largest and most-seen organ. From the cracks on the sides of your mouth, to the spots on your back, the hard skin on your feet, the dry skin on your scalp or the pimples on the backs of your arms – they all add to the insecurities that we show the outside world. But if you think of these imperfections as *perfect* imperfections you can change your perception and look at the positive colours of the skin.

So whether you are having a bad skin day or a good skin day, start the day in a positive way with this facial exercise below.

Action: Start the day with some facial gymnastics to get the blood flowing around the face. Start by pretending to chew a toffee for a minute, then open your mouth for 10 seconds as wide as you can and repeat three times. Then stretch your neck to the right and left, front and back, holding for 10 seconds in each direction. This way you will open up your third eye chakra, which is the centre for intuition and foresight and is driven by the principle of openness and imagination. It will also open your crown chakra, which gives us access to a higher state of consciousness.

The emotional body

The emotional effect of skin conditions can be tough. From being bullied in the classroom at primary school to being embarrassed in front of the opposite sex, these experiences at a young age can instil feelings of insecurity and imperfection and create emotional scars that shape our character and future life. Recognising the emotional effects of this on sufferers is integral to managing and preventing further imbalance. Remember that confidence comes from within you, it makes you stronger. Having to go through tough times can build a greater resilience and understanding of 'self' as you get older.

Action: If you had issues with your skin when you were younger, or still have them now, reach out to close friends and family members with whom you can talk openly about your feelings. Do not let these feelings fester inside as they will build up and turn into something else.

The nutritional body

The results of eating good food will last longer than a facelift.

Your food and lifestyle choices all have an impact on the appearance of your skin. Avoid excessive levels of sugar, caffeine and junk food as well as smoking and alcohol and make a note of the changes this makes to your skin. There is no better treatment for the body than good organic seasonal food prepared by your own hands for anti-ageing.

Great food with which to feed your skin

Almonds: These nuts are so versatile and they help fight the assaults of life such as pollution, toxins and processed foods. You can use them in your cooking; to make salads; in smoothies; and on your skin. Almonds have stacks of vitamin E, which is a fat-soluble vitamin that protects and heals the skin. For example, it's been shown to be beneficial for dry skin sufferers, and it's also great for anti-ageing.

Tomatoes: The natural sun protection factor – tomatoes contain an antioxidant called lycopene, so by eating a diet containing tomatoes you can support your skin's natural SPF levels, protecting you from the sun.

Coconut oil: You can use this oil in your cooking and baking and directly on your skin as a moisturiser – a double whammy! Top tip: add it to smoothies to get a good source of fuel that smoothies are often deficient in.

Action: Keep a food/skin diary and pay attention to which foods in your diet cause reactions. A food diary is a great tool for highlighting what works for your body and what doesn't. Make a note of the time you consumed the foods or liquids and then note 1–2 hours later how you are feeling.

Food / mood / bowel diary record (7 days)

Please indicate the quantity of food and the method of preparation (i.e. steamed, grilled, poached, fried, or baked).

Item	Day 1	Day 2	Day 3	Day 4	Day 5	Day 6	Day 7
Breakfast							
Feeling							
Mid-morning							
Lunch							
Feeling							
Mid-afternoon							
Dinner							
Feeling							
Bedtime							
Feeling							

Item	Day 1	Day 2	Day 3	Day 4	Day 5	Day 6	Day 7
Snacks mid-morning and afternoon							
Liquids (water, tea, coffee, juice)							
Bowel movements (no., time, consistency)							
Movement							

The physical body

The personal care product industry makes billions of pounds each year and is still growing. It is also a fairly unregulated industry. However, new guidance from the government website for organic labelling states that for a product to be organic, 95 per cent of the ingredients have to be organic.[2] This is great news as it means we can be sure of the provenance of what we are putting on our skin.

The skin is tough and robust but that doesn't mean you don't need to look after it on the outside as well as the inside. Take some time to think about all the beauty products in your bathroom and the cleaning products in your kitchen. How many of these come into daily contact with your skin? Look at the labels – how many harmful chemicals are you putting on your skin every day?

Ask yourself before you went to work this morning how many beauty products did your skin come into contact with? Did you use toothpaste, perfume, skin serum, lip salve, shaving balm? For women in particular it is estimated that on average they will use over 200 chemicals on their skin daily and around 60 per cent of these get absorbed directly into the bloodstream.

A study detected lead in 61 per cent of the 33 lipsticks tested, with levels ranging from 0.03 to 0.65 parts per million, yet experts say there is no safe level of lead in the blood.[3] Think about how many times you may reapply your lipstick or kiss your girlfriend/boyfriend who is wearing some.[4] You could be ingesting up to 87 milligrams of lead a day and other heavy metals from lip glosses, too.

The great news is that there is a whole array of beauty companies and household product companies that do not use any chemicals or nasties. Here are some of my favourites:

Beauty products

The companies below have good sites from which you can purchase natural beauty products.

- Content Beauty and Wellbeing; www.contentbeautywellbeing.com
- Neal's Yard Remedies; www.nealsyardremedies.com
- Green People; www.greenpeople.co.uk
- Natracare; www.natracare.com.
- Antipodes; http://antipodesnature.com
- Plant Me Botanics; http://plantmebotanics.com

Household products

- Dr Bronner's Castile household cleaning soap; www.drbronner.co.uk
- Attitude Living; www.attitudeliving.com
- Ecover Zero; www.ecoverdirect.com

Top tip:

A combination of lemon juice, bicarbonate of soda and vinegar makes a really effective way to clean your house – and it is cheap, too. Cut a lemon in half, and dip the cut side in a paste of bicarbonate of soda and vinegar to scrub your surfaces clean. Check out this link for ways to clean your house without the chemical eruption: https://www.thespruce.com/homemade-and-natural-cleaning-products-1900456

In the table below I have put together some of the most common synthetic chemicals to avoid that are found in our beauty and household products.[5]

You might also want to check out this website, which has a lot more info on what to look out for: http://www.ewg.org/skindeep/#.Wp7CciOcY0o

Which products should you avoid?

Chemical ingredient to avoid	Found in ...	Alternative
Propylene glycol Also known as PPG and PEG. The Food and Drug Administration (FDA) requires protective clothing to be worn when the skin is in contact with this product	Some deodorants and antiperspirants	Salt rock deodorant
Sodium laureth sulfate A common foaming agent that can cause irritation to the skin and the eyes	Most shampoos and conditioners, soaps	Castile soap, yucca extract, soapwort
Phthalates A group of chemicals used to make plastics more flexible and harder to break. Some phthalates are used as solvents (dissolving agents) for other materials such as nail polish. Phthalates will disrupt your endocrine system, especially oestrogen and organs such as the liver, kidneys[6] and lungs	As a primary source, all plastics; as a secondary source, all foods that have been through factory-type scenarios, nail polish	Bio-based plastics[7] – which you can tell by the label
Parabens Used as a preservative. Linked to cancer, endocrine disruption and reproductive toxicity	Many products for the bathroom and kitchen, so make sure you use your marigolds	Natural preservatives; always choose a product that states it is 'paraben free'

So, as pretty as the packaging is and as enticing as the advertising campaigns say these products are, you will be exponentially better off internally and externally without any of the chemicals listed above in your system.

Throw things out: Take a paper bag and empty your shelves and cupboards of the lotions you have been hoarding since your school days. Empty the products if you can and recycle the plastic after washing the containers clean. Then make a vow to yourself to buy fewer products, and to make sure they are ecologically sound. The last time I checked, a bar of soap did the same as a plastic hand dispenser filled with soap! Not only are you being savvy in the finances, but you are being environmentally responsible, too, and you'll have brighter, happier skin to show for it!

HOW TO LOOK AFTER YOUR SKIN

Your skin will love you if you feed it with water, which is the simplest way to look after it. You might be surprised at what a difference this simple step can make. Clients of mine who make a concerted effort to drink more water find their skin glows and they are less prone to oily patches and breakouts or acne.

Here are some pointers to improve the look and feel of your skin. By feeding your skin from the inside you can reduce inflammation and hold off ageing for as long as possible.

First, look out for signs that your skin is under stress, such as:

Dry skin: When you are stressed you produce more cortisol, which inhibits your body's ability to hold on to water, leaving it looking dry.

Acne/spotty skin: This for women can be down to hormonal changes but also down to the food you eat. So reduce the high-sugar foods and the caffeine (which dries the skin) and add more water and hydrating foods such as cucumbers and coconut water.

Redness on the cheeks: This broken capillary look can be due to low hydrochloric acid levels, which can decrease during stressful periods.

How to keep your skin looking youthful

When it comes to anti-ageing, there are many factors you can avoid, which will help your skin to stay healthy, including:

- smoking
- drinking enough unfiltered water
- breathing polluted air
- lack of movement
- eating refined and processed foods
- using beauty products full of chemicals
- overuse of make-up and perfumes
- negative thoughts and resentment

While you can look to supplements, non-invasive medical procedures and expensive creams to keep you looking youthful, there is no substitute for good food, plenty of water, exercise and sleep. It has been proven that living a healthy life has a longer shelf life than any medical procedure, facial, peel, acid peel or anything that involves a needle, and all you need is some motivation to get started!

The majority of diseases that we have to contend with these days are more preventable than you may think. Cancers, diabetes, obesity and cardiovascular diseases are all the result of lifestyles that allow your cells to go and turn off your anti-ageing genes. By switching from lifestyle factors that cause disease to those that prevent it you can help reverse the ageing of your cells and so reduce the risk of illness.

The environment we live in causes cells to age; we have never before been exposed to so many chemicals – in our food, on our plants and in our animals. Bill Wilcox, founder of Healthexcel Metabolic Typing, talks about the importance of efficient digestion. He says if you are unable to convert the food you eat into energy, you will not be able to meet your genetically based requirements. To do this, you need healthy cells to create healthy organ systems.[8]

Good foods to keep skin youthful

Meals and snacks	Nutrition	Benefits
On waking in the morning	Cold-pressed ginger root, turmeric root, and lemon and lemon rind with cold or hot water	Reduces inflammation and mops up free radicals that prematurely age you
First meal of the day	Red pepper baked with a duck egg, spinach and anchovies, and tomatoes drizzled with basil oil and walnuts	Bursting with vitamin C and good omega fats for healthy-looking skin
Snack, if desired	Carrot juice with ginger, apple and beetroot	High in anti-fungal properties
Second meal of the day	Salmon fillet, steamed with kohlrabi, leeks and kale, served with garlic and garden herbs	Salmon is full of omega 3 which keeps the skin elastic and plump
Snack	Apple slices and nut butter	Satisfying, good fats
Third meal of the day	Green vegetables (Tenderstem broccoli, green peppers, beansprouts, courgettes, spinach), stir-fried with ginger root, chilli and prawns with a side of kimchi	Rebalances the microbiome and good bacteria
Bedtime snack / activity	Cinnamon and chamomile tea	Calming effect to promote sleep

Rose for the skin

The rose aroma is best known for its calming and balancing effects, and is particularly beneficial for dry, sensitive or ageing skins. It provides a soothing and astringent effect which helps diminish redness and skin irritation.

The seeds of the plants are called rosehips and contain vitamins A, B3, C, D and E, as well as essential fatty acids, which are particularly beneficial for the skin as they quickly absorb into the skin to help with tissue regeneration. Rosehip oil contains trans-retinoic acid, which aids in skin regeneration and helps reduce fine lines and wrinkles.

My favourite is Organic Rose Otto serum by Plant Me Botanics[9]; part of a range of 320 MHz bio-energetic beauty treatments inspired by ancient botanicals. These products are blissfully committed to no additives or synthetic perfume, fragrance, parabens, PEGs or animal testing. They are also vegan and suitable for all skin types.

PATHOLOGIES OF THE SKIN

Free radicals are like single-winged aeroplanes careering around your body causing damage by crashing into your sides, unable to stay in a straight flight path through the arteries and intestines! The more damage that this plane causes, the more inflammation occurs to the tissues of the body, unless the Red Cross get sent to the crash site soon to start repairing the damage. In this case, the Red Cross equals antioxidants and they enter the body essentially disguised as fruit and vegetables.

However, when antioxidants don't jump in to repair the cellular DNA membranes, the transformation of healthy happy cells leads to diseased or dying cells. This process is the inflammation which is well cited as being the etiology of all disease (as you will see in psoriasis and eczema below), but the great news is that it is largely preventable and can be managed through targeted nutrition and lifestyle choices. Inflammation comes from the Latin word *inflammo*, meaning I set alight, which may be exactly what the surface of the skin feels like to sufferers. Inflammation is part of the body's immune response; initially it is beneficial for when the body experiences pain, signalling to your body that something is wrong and the tissues need protection. It is also a process by which white blood cells are produced to protect the body from an infection or a foreign organism, such as bacteria and viruses.

Psoriasis

Psoriasis is an auto-immune disease in which the epidermal cells of the skin are produced too fast without complete maturation, creating visible hallmarks including shiny silvery scales, pitting of the nails, red markings and patches all over the body. It is not an uncommon skin condition to see flare up on the skin at any age and there are many reasons why it presents itself.

If inflammation is present the immune system will be under attack. Inflammation can start by a bacterial infection or food allergies and the typical signs are swelling, redness and heat to the infected area, where there will also be pain and a loss of function. In that area the blood vessels dilate, reducing blood pressure and allowing more blood to get to the area. At the heart of lots of skin conditions there is a redness or raised look to the skin (which is inflammation) and here the treatment is multifactorial.

Types of psoriasis

There are many different types of psoriasis and all have varying treatment programmes:

- **Plaque psoriasis** (also called psoriasis vulgaris) is the most common form, most often affecting the scalp, knees, elbows and lower back, and causes nail pitting. It appears as raised skin with red patches, covered with a silvery white build-up of dead skin cells or scale. The itchy, painful patches can crack and bleed.
- **Guttate psoriasis** often begins in childhood or young adulthood and is the second most common type of psoriasis. It presents as red paint patches all over the body, but not on the face, and a streptococcal throat infection that causes a systemic infection and leaves the body after three or so months.
- **Inverse psoriasis**, also known as intertriginous psoriasis, causes red lesions in folds of the body that may look smooth and shiny; they can occur on the genitals or areas near the genitals, such as the upper thighs and groin. It's common for people with inverse psoriasis to have another type of psoriasis somewhere else on their body at the same time.
- **Pustular psoriasis** causes white blisters of pus that surround red skin. The pus consists of white blood cells. When pus-filled bumps cover the body, you may have bright-red skin and feel ill, exhausted, have a fever, chills, severe itching, rapid pulse, loss of appetite or muscle weakness.
- **Erythrodermic psoriasis** is a dangerous and rare form of the disease, characterised by a widespread, fiery redness and exfoliation of the skin that causes severe itching and pain. This type of psoriasis occurs in 3 per cent of people with psoriasis, according to the National Psoriasis Foundation (NPF).

Reasons why psoriasis may occur

The inflammatory reasons why psoriasis might occur are vast and in most cases they will be multi-faceted. A lack of sleep, a chronic stress response, UV light, chemicals, alcohol abuse, stress, lithium, anti-malarial medication and beta blockers have all played a part in this inflammatory condition, to name just a few factors. Non-alcoholic fatty liver disease has also been linked to psoriasis in various research papers.

Useful measures to counteract the effects of psoriasis

Fish oils: Foods high in fish oils have been proven to benefit people suffering from psoriasis. Omega 3 fatty acids have a direct correlation to inflammatory biomarkers, namely inflammatory cytokines, which are proteins that send signals that inflammation is present in the body.[10]

Look after your gut: The relationship between the gut and your skin is huge. When the defence systems are down you can get infections of pathogens, unwanted bacteria or an overgrowth of yeast and fungi. If these are plaguing your gut you are likely to have a leaky gut, a less diverse microbiome and your risk of psoriasis will be greater. The gut is our second skin and tells a story of what is happening on the inside. So if you do have skin issues, cleaning up the gut is not a bad idea, and has health benefits to boot.

Eat the right foods: Not all foods are created equally. Some foods create inflammation for one person but not the next. You can find this out by doing a food intolerance test or by eliminating the foods that you have isolated as responsible for creating unwanted reactions. Often foods high in salicylates (mushrooms, aubergines, courgettes) and histamine food (champagne, fermented foods, cured meats) can create inflammation, as can nightshade foods (tomatoes, peppers, potatoes).

Cinnamon and honey mask: Mix together 2 tablespoons of raw organic honey, 1 teaspoon of coconut oil and ½ teaspoon of ground cinnamon. Smooth the mixture over the face, keeping it away from the eyes, as the cinnamon can be an irritant. Relax for 5–10 minutes then gently remove the mask with a damp cloth. Honey and cinnamon used together helps to fight inflammation because of the anti-inflammatory, antioxidant and antibacterial properties. Add a couple of drops of tea tree oil to the mask above during an active acne breakout.

Take vitamins and minerals: Vitamin D[11] and vitamin A[12] help to inhibit the formation of polyamines, which are toxins found in higher levels in people with psoriasis. Vitamin D is a fat-soluble vitamin which can be harnessed from many animal products and through exposure to the sun. The recommended daily intake in the UK is 400–800 international units (IU). Vitamin A (the most beneficial vitamin when treating the skin in general) is a fat-soluble vitamin otherwise known as retinol, and is converted from beta carotene in plants. The current recommended daily value for vitamin A is 5,000 IU, and it can be found in carrots, red peppers, spinach, tomatoes and squash, to name a few food sources.

Chondroitin sulfate: This is found around the joints of the body and is typically used for healing. Most sources for human consumption are from cow or shark cartilage.[13] In one study carried out by Verges et al, in 2005, patients were given 800mg of chondroitin sulfate for two months. The results were majoritively positive – all but one patient saw a big improvement in swelling, redness, flaking and itching (all symptoms of psoriasis).

Sarsaparilla: Native to North and South America, this is claimed to 'attack and neutralise toxins in the blood' and has been used for skin conditions such as psoriasis for centuries. Take half to one cup of a standard root decoction 2–3 times daily. Alternatively, take 1–2g of root powder in tablets or capsules twice daily or 2–3ml of a standard tincture or fluid extract twice daily. You can get these from a reputable health food shop.

Tea tree oil: The tea tree produces an oil that is said to have antiseptic qualities. It has been used in everything from dentistry to dermatology and may be particularly helpful to sufferers of scalp psoriasis. However, it can cause allergic reactions in some individuals and should be used with care. Additionally, no clinical studies have examined the effectiveness of tea tree oil in the treatment of psoriasis.

Quercetin: Is a flavonoid antioxidant found in plant foods and has been reported to effectively fight inflammatory-type conditions such as psoriasis. It is found in foods such as apples, peppers, red wine and dark berries!

Eczema or atopic dermatitis

The word eczema is derived from the Greek word for 'boiling'; it is a chronic ongoing condition of the skin that can flare up for many reasons. The skin becomes flaky, inflamed and can ooze; there is also a thickening of the skin and vesiculation (small sacs containing liquid from blisters). There are many different types of eczema – atopic, contact (irritant and allergen – ACD), adult and infantile seborrhoeic, discoid, pompholyx, asteatotic, varicose – and you should get a diagnosis from a doctor so that you know what type you are dealing with. It is worth noting that eczema and dermatitis are interchangeable. Unlike psoriasis, eczema is not an auto-immune condition and is not characterised by silvery scaly skin, but what is similar about both conditions is the need for good gut health to counteract them. As Hippocrates said, all disease starts in the gut.

As the condition becomes self-perpetuating – one itch, two itches, then three itches more – the skin becomes torn and starts to bleed, so for this reason alone sufferers should wear cotton mitts at night to reduce scarring. A short-term solution is found in a cooling pain-relieving cream, which will provide some relief but does not get to the root cause of the issue.

Reasons why eczema may occur and what it might look like for you
Eczema is characterised, as many skin conditions are, by redness, itching and oozing. The best solution for skin conditions is not to scratch, which is easier said than done. No one is exempt from eczema

at any time in his or her life; from babies to adults, for a plethora of reasons, eczema can develop – heat, bacterial skin infections, dust, animal hair, pollen, perfumed creams, colourings, moulds, clothing, stress and humidity can all play a part. Below are more symptoms of the root cause of eczema.

Genetic predisposition: A genetic predisposition or a deficiency in the filaggrin gene is now thought to lead to atopic eczema. The majority of us will have this gene but people with atopic eczema have filaggrin loss-of-function mutations.[14]

Food allergies and intolerances: It has been found that people with eczema will have high levels of IgE, secretory IgA[15] (Sig A) and eosinophils. High levels of IgE simply mean certain foods trigger this response, including eggs, shellfish, wheat, cow's milk, soy and nuts (a food allergy and an intolerance are not the same; an allergy is an abnormal reaction of the immune system and an intolerance is when you have trouble digesting the food). Sig A is an antibody protein that is secreted into the body from the gastrointestinal tract to provide the first line of defence against unwanted pathogens. Sig A is a bit like a wall around a fort; if the wall is intact no invaders/pathogens can get in and if the defences are low the wall is broken, then pathogens can get in. Eosinophils are disease-fighting white blood cells that more often than not indicate a parasite infection, infection and/or inflammation.

Low HCL: Hydrochloric acid breaks down protein in the stomach where the pH of the stomach should be around 0.8–1.5 (see stomach chapter). While excess levels of HCL are often blamed for the cause of many health problems it is worth noting that when under stress HCL levels are one of the first things to deplete. Conditions such as diabetes, insulin resistance, childhood asthma, depression and fatigue are all symptomatic of HCL levels being low. Essentially, when low acid is present, food is not broken down efficiently, pathogens can get into the body via the stomach if you eat or drink infected water or food, and these factors contribute to absorption and digestive issues, food intolerances and all play out on the skin.

Sluggish liver function: The liver detoxifies all the toxins you take into the body and excretes them in a water-soluble form via the kidneys, bile and the intestines. So if your liver function is impaired you run the risk of these toxins being recirculated around the body, causing fatigue and absorption, digestion and elimination problems. Elimination problems will show up on the skin as inflammation that has been created in the body and it must find another way to be excreted.

Healing options for eczema

Often with eczema both allopathic and alternative healing options are used because the condition can be so unpleasant and irritating. Steroid cream often solves the problem temporarily, but the condition has the potential to come back if you do not change anything else in your life, such as your diet and lifestyle. The skin can often become as fragile as a paper ship after years of using a cream, especially on the inner elbows, and this often triggers an investigation into natural ways of healing. There are over 100 different drugs given for dermatitis conditions, which will either be an emollient (moisturiser) or a corticosteroid (hormones). It is always up to you which method you decide to treat your condition with.

Here are some other options to try in order to avoid those steroid creams:

Bathing in magnesium bath salts: This not only improves skin barrier function but also enhances skin hydration and reduces inflammation in atopic eczema and dry skin. It has favourable effects on inflammatory diseases and bouts of stress, too.

Test for bacteria: Eczema is often aggravated by bacteria called *Staphylococcus aureus*, which can slow down the skin's healing process. This can be tested for via the urine and can be cleared up naturally with the use of antibacterial herbs such as allicin, oregano or antimicrobial silver therapy.

Apply a soothing herb: Aloe vera is a plant with a gel-like substance inside its spikes which offers antimicrobial properties and can help heal skin and manage eczema when applied topically. It is recommended you apply the gel twice a day to soothe a flare-up.

Eating for skin conditions

Freshness, quality and seasonality all contribute to how your skin looks and how your skin tissue behaves. Nutritionally dense foods will encourage your skin to be bright and fresh, processed food and high-sugar foods can contribute to dull-looking skin.

Foods to avoid if you have eczema, psoriasis or other skin conditions

Pro-inflammatory foods	Reason	Alternative / substitute
Food additives and preservatives – MSG, aspartame, food dyes	Often triggers of inflammation in people who are already experiencing inflammatory conditions such as arthritis and colitis	Beetroot is a natural preservative for meats Watch out for labels that include preservatives
Processed meats often high in saturated and trans fats	Processed meats are classed as a carcinogenic, meaning that they promote cancer growth	Buy organic meat from locally sourced butchers and farmers, in keeping with the seasons
Refined sugars (white, brown and cane sugar)	Decreases immunity and contributes to overall inflammation in the body	Raw honey, Canadian maple syrup, cinnamon

High omega 6 fatty acids (safflower, sunflower, soya bean, corn oil) vegetable oil	Leads to inflammation, contributing to many health problems and diseases	Coconut oil, olive oil and raw grass-fed butter
Dairy products, especially cow's	Contains proteins that are common allergens and that trigger inflammatory responses (constipation, diarrhoea, rash) in sensitive individuals	Nut milks that are organic, cold-pressed and unsweetened
Alcohol	Irritates the stomach lining and puts stress on the liver, which in turn can create an imbalance in hormones and cause your skin to flare up	Angostura bitters/tequila. Bitters are a great way to up your digestion powers and it looks like an alcoholic drink. Tequila is one of the purest alcohols available, so your body can break it down more efficiently

Superfoods for skin conditions

Colostrum: This has been proven to naturally support and restore balance to the immune system. The best source of colostrum is bovine (cow) because it has very high levels of immunoglobulin G (IgG), a natural antibody that provides systemic immunity. It plays a role in sealing the gut which in turn supports the immune system and improves the make-up of your skin. You can get this in liquid form. My favourite is Liquid Gold by OraMune.

Green tea: This has been considered a health tonic all over the world for centuries but especially among ezcema sufferers as it has been shown to reduce inflammation and itching. Two active green tea extracts are catechins and L-theanine. Catechins such as epigallocatechin gallate are the most active ingredient in green tea; it is an antioxidant reported to be a hundred times more potent than vitamin C and 25 times more potent than vitamin E in protecting against free-radical attack.

Alpha lipoic acid: A potent antioxidant that helps to maintain mito-chondrial health and inhibit skin-damaging inflammation and free radicals that is found in our bodies. You can take it in through many food sources, too, such as broccoli, spinach, red meat, organ meat, Brussels sprouts, rice bran and yams.

Case study

Eczema and acne

I met Thomas on what felt like a lazy afternoon, or perhaps it was just his mood that was catching. There seemed to be a fog of fatigue following him around and every now and then I felt I had to ask if he was still with me, to which he'd reply, 'Sorry, just zoned out.' Maybe, I thought, it was just a teenage thing. Thomas presented with extreme fatigue but also with eczema, acne and bouts of the blues. He itched a lot and talked even more.

He was interesting, smart and obviously intelligent, with a modern, music composer's brain, hyped on ideas and technology – hence the rapid-fire talking. His autonomic nervous system was on overdrive and his symptoms began to paint their own picture. On waking, he admitted to still feeling half-asleep. With his scalp irritating him all the time he took a steroid cream, but he hoped there might be better ways to treat his condition. He'd been referred on from a CBT therapist, who'd been treating him for anxiety and depression.

Anything that presents on the skin is the body's way of pointing out there's another organ or organ system that's out of balance. Looking to reason with the brain/mind isn't the answer;

90 per cent of serotonin, the happy hormone, is created in the gastrointestinal tract, so that's the logical place to start investigating. I spent some time explaining the workings of the gut and suggesting immediate changes to his diet and lifestyle. I reassured him it wouldn't be forever and in two weeks we'd be able to see what was working and what wasn't. I suggested if he did nothing else that he should remove 100 per cent gluten and dairy products from his diet and reduce his consumption of alcohol. Removing dairy and gluten offers a chance not only to reduce inflammation in the gut but also to eat other foods and thereby increase the diversity of the microbiome, get creative in the kitchen and eat more seasonally. I also asked him to drink bone broth, cold-press juices and more water every day.

At our second meeting, I almost didn't recognise him, he practically skipped into the room. His skin was no longer so high-maintenance and the fatigue had lifted dramatically, as had the morning fog. His face was clearer and his skin was not as dry after showering – a complication of eczema being that water cannot be locked in, and this lack of moisture leads to tightness and itching.

Thomas was finding the suggested diet manageable, although, as he pointed out, you don't miss something until you know you can't have it and then you realise gluten, dairy and alcohol are in almost everything you eat. And of course he'd put an astute finger on the truth: we're probably all eating foods to which we're intolerant without realising it.

He said he was happy to continue with the regime of increased vegetables and also told me he juiced, sometimes four times a day, was that OK? I refrained from giving him a high five and assured him it was like a beneficial intravenous shot straight into the body. He also told me that when drinking beer he was getting hot flushes and, as we both agreed, this was unlikely to be the menopause, so I prescribed him champagne of the highest quality, which he felt was something he could live with. Champagne, along with tequila, is a purer form of alcohol than the majority available and therefore easier for the body to process. Another issue he had was with mucus that couldn't be dislodged without harsh coughing. I prescribed 100ml (3½ fl oz) of broccoli juice and 100ml (3½ fl oz) of cabbage juice daily on rotation for the next six weeks, because these contain sulforaphane, which reduces inflammation, and glutamine, which helps heal the gastrointestinal lining.

A month later I received an email from Thomas:

Dear Hannah,
Just to give you an update, all is still going pretty much on schedule apart from slip-ups when staying with friends, like I had some pizza the other day, which was silly. I also have the odd drop of milk in tea. Skin is feeling and looking so much better, quite a lot of people noticing, which is nice, and motivates you to carry on doing it.
Thanks, my favourite lifestyle coach,
Best wishes,
T-Rob

STRESS AND THE SKIN

You could say that stress is anything that poses a threat to our wellbeing. However, stress is not all bad, because we need stress to keep moving! Our fight-or-flight response is our body's sympathetic nervous system reacting to a stressful event. Our body produces larger quantities of the chemicals cortisol, adrenaline and noradrenaline, which trigger a higher heart rate, heightened muscle preparedness, sweating and alertness – all these factors help us protect ourselves in a dangerous or challenging situation. But when we are in fight-or-flight response mode all non-essential body functions slow down, such as our digestive and immune systems, so that all resources can be concentrated on rapid breathing, blood flow, alertness and muscle use.

So how does this affect the skin? The hormones produced when we are stressed – adrenaline, cortisol and DHEA – can cause all sorts of physiological imbalances.

- Stress can cause your skin to produce more oil (sebum) which leads to clogged pores and the appearance of whiteheads and blackheads.
- Stress decreases the immune system, which lives in your gut, and impairs the body's ability to heal and fight infections.
- If you already have skin problems, stress can make them worse as stress promotes inflammation and your preexisting conditions like acne, eczema, rosacea and psoriasis can flare up.
- Stress can cause your skin to become dehydrated as the lipid barrier function decreases. This keeps our skin moist and youthful.
- And lastly stress can really age us. When we are stressed our hormones, hydration, food choices, movement all start to change, usually for the worse, and this challenges the cell turnover and collagen production, leading to fine lines, acne, blemished and tired-looking skin.

Stress is the modern-day nemesis that is impossible to escape – especially if you live in a city. To help combat stress or at least be able to deal with it more efficiently you should try to add some me-time into your day, but think carefully about how you will spend this time. Often my really stressed-out clients add more stress to their lives by signing up to eight-week mindfulness courses and yoga lessons

– these are the people who can't bear to be in their own company for more than five minutes doing nothing, so they struggle to do even a minute of quiet self-reflection. I am a big fan of mindfulness but if you use it like a pill you will not get the desired result.

There are different types of quiet and rest and some people can achieve it more naturally than others. The optimal rest we get is the time when we are in bed asleep. Ideally, you should be asleep before midnight to rest physically and psychologically. According to the circadian rhythms (sleep cycle) the body repairs itself physically between the hours of 10pm and 2am and then physiologically until 6am. So if you get into bed after midnight you can feel exhausted physically on waking. Then we have other rest periods when we are doing things for ourselves, like enjoying our hobbies and spending some time in our own company with our thoughts. If you have a monkey mind – a mind that cannot stay still and focus – this is a hard place to be, so you may always find yourself with the TV or stereo on so you don't hear the thoughts. Changing your ways takes time, but making a start or becoming aware that you find it difficult to be in your own space is the first step to mindfulness.

Try a few of these options to find some calm:

- Read a book line by line without losing the story. If you do, go back to the beginning.
- Sit and focus on your breath and count to 100.
- Walk up and down the garden bare-footed and hum as you go.
- Turn off all the electronics (radio, music, TV, laptop) in your house and listen to the silence for 10 minutes.

Case study

Twenty-first-century stress: psoriasis

Elizabeth has skin like a porcelain doll, with rarely a blemish or a spot to fight with, much to the envy of her female friends, I'm sure. However, in times of stress she started to get these red bumps, specifically on her lower legs and tummy. Initially I suspected follicular dermatitis. I recommended that she see a nurse specialising in psoriasis. She was able to give Elizabeth some medical advice as well as alternative treatments, giving her a clearer picture of how long it would stay around. This gave Elizabeth the peace of mind that clients often need when symptoms arise. We cannot be experts in every condition and so a strong referral is vital for the wellbeing of the client. Elizabeth was in media, working long hours and on an often sensitive, traumatic, emotional and all-encompassing subject. When she was involved in a project it took all of her, probably more than she was aware, and this was starting to affect her health. Often in a world all of her own, her health started to take a back seat as her energy was invested emotionally and physically in the events and people she was working with and for.

People have coping mechanisms when stress occurs; some go for a run, some box, some overeat, some undereat – Elizabeth smoked pot, but coupled with alcohol, coffee and late nights, her body was saying give me a break. She had done this for 15 years and not been without alcohol for over a month in adulthood – only abstaining in January. This abuse was showing on her skin. I always remind clients that symptoms are at the end of the pathology model, not at the beginning. A lot of dysfunction has to go on before the symptom arises. Just think about an iceberg peeking out of the water; it's not until you see the size of the iceberg underneath the water level that you see the scale of the problem.

Psoriasis can flare up when people are stressed. On an adrenal stress profile test, Elizabeth's cortisol levels were low, signifying that she has been in a state of stress for some time, which fitted with everything she was saying to me. Her ability to cope with all the demands of the job she was experiencing was taking its toll. When she was on holiday or simply not on a contract job of long hours and late nights there were no signs of psoriasis. Sometimes you find that it's the lifestyle factors that need addressing the most and this was the case with Elizabeth. She had got to a place where her job was causing her to self-medicate with pot and alcohol to cope with the stress of it, which spiralled into late nights, not enough repair or rest. If stress has become part of your life, other symptoms, like digestive complaints, fall into insignificance and you become less sensitive to them as you just keep doing what you are doing, albeit not very well and with little energy.

It is just as important to find the root cause of what is causing an illness – in this case the stress – and deal with that, rather than just treating the outward symptoms.

TOP 10 TIPS FOR HEALTHY-LOOKING SKIN

1   **Hydration:** My first rule of thumb is to drink as soon as you wake up, because you have just had a good eight hours in bed asleep (ideally) and the body's breakfast should always be some silky-smooth filtered water to feed those cells at the start of the day. Drink before each meal, though, as drinking too much water in between can interfere with the digestive enzymes and their ability to break

down food efficiently. Also drink water after every bowel movement, as it aids peristalsis and elimination can leave your bowel dry.

2. **Broccoli:** The powerhouse of DNA protection. Juice it, cook it, steam it, eat it raw or even rub it on your skin – it doesn't really matter how you take it because broccoli is your lifeline. You must have a relationship with this vegetable because it is the superhero of the vegetable world; broccoli has the ability to save lives! Sulforaphane is the dietary component of broccoli that repairs the damaged DNA, or the damaged stem cells, and prevents the cells going rogue in the first place.

3 **Juice turmeric:** I love to juice this but I also like to add it to cooking meats and fish, not only for its colour but also for its anti-inflammatory and antioxidant properties. It has the propensity to stain the skin and most things it comes into contact with, so wear gloves when handling the root or you will stain your nails and hands and all kitchen surfaces.

4 **Chop carrots:** Did your parents ever tell you to eat carrots because they'll make you see in the dark? Well, that's because vitamin A is found in carrots: this vitamin is converted in plants from beta carotene and helps prevent a condition called night blindness, as well as giving you healthy-looking skin. Vitamin A is a valuable key to flawless and young-looking skin, so make sure you eat those carrots.

5 Take vitamin D: Unless you get outside every day and see the sun, your vitamin D levels will be low and a supplement is a very common prescription now. Vitamin D is vital for the skin's cell growth and metabolism. It supports the body's immune system and helps prevent free radical damage. The NHS suggests adults and children over the age of five should take a 10mcg supplement between October and mid-March.[16]

6 **Decrease alcohol consumption:** Within eight minutes of drinking three 25ml shots of vodka your carotenoid antioxidant levels in the skin drop dramatically, and when these levels drop your skin essentially

ages. The breakdown products of alcohol produce excessive amounts of free radicals, i.e. alcohol that damages the skin; this doubles if you are drinking in the sun.

7   **Reduce sun exposure:** The most common type of cancer is skin cancer, primarily because of the UV rays that our bodies are not protected from. So if you are in the sun, make sure that you are wearing an organic sunscreen. I love the scent-free factor 30 by Green People.

8   **Sleep:** The skin's best friend. People who sleep for the recommended eight hours a night without waking up with stress or anxiety or needing to pee will have a greater chance of staying younger for longer. Be in bed and asleep without your phone before midnight and you'll be on your way to better skin.

9   **Snack on almonds:** More than a handful of almonds is excessive, so take just that amount and move out of the kitchen! I love almonds as they are a great source of magnesium and vitamin E, which help cells produce energy and protein. Magnesium is believed to counter the effects of the stress hormones that can make you age faster and exacerbate skin conditions. Homemade almond milk is ideal as a tonic for the skin, provided you like the taste.

10 **Use paraben-free products:** A paraben is a chemical that is used as a preservative. Now that you know a lot more about your skin you will remember that your body's second mouth is your skin, so anything you put on your skin – from the water in the bath tub to the scented moisturiser that came free with your perfume – your body has to deal with. So stop, bin it and use something organic and natural or nothing. I love Green People and Antipode – both natural and organic skincare ranges and as essential as your underwear. Never go without it! Start the day with a cold shower and then warm up with some beautiful organic products.

Footnotes

(1) Kushi, M., *Your Body Never Lies* (New York, 2007).

(2) Defra, 'Organic Food Labelling Rules', www.gov.uk/guidance/organic-food-labelling-rules (accessed on 21/01/2016).

(3) CDC, 'National Biomonitoring Program', www.cdc.gov/biomonitoring/Lead_FactSheet.html (accessed on 21/01/2016).

(4) FDA, 'Limiting lead in lipsticks and other cosmetics', www.fda.gov/cosmetics/productsingredients/potentialcontaminants/ucm137 224.htm (accessed on 21/01/2016).

(5) Campaign for Safe Cosmetics, 'Phthalates', www.safecosmetics.org/get-the-facts/chemicals-of-concern/phthalates/#sthash.IRr7FMN1.dpuf (accessed on 21/01/2016).

(6) Kataria, A., Trasande, L., Trachtman, H., 'The effects of environmental chemicals on renal function', *Nature Reviews Nephrology* 11(10) (London, 2015).

(7) 'How to dispose of bio-based plastics', www.allthings.bio/dispose-bio-based-plastics/ (accessed on 21/01/2016).

(8) 'What is an organ system – Definition & Pictures', study.com/academy/lesson/what-is-an-organ-system-definition-pictures-quiz.html (accessed on 21/06/2016).

(9) Bio-energetic Skincare, plantmebotanics.com (accessed on 21/01/2016).

(10) Zhang, J.-M., 'Cytokines, Inflammation and Pain', *International Anesthesiology Clinics* (2007).

(11) Balato, A. et al, 'Interleukin-1 family members are enhanced in psoriasis and suppressed by vitamin D and retinoic acid', *Archives of Dermatological Research* (Berlin, 2013).

(12) Chapman, M.S., 'Vitamin A: history, current uses, and controversies', *Seminars in Cutaneous Medicine and Surgery* (2012).

(13) Verges, J. et al, 'Clinical and histopathological improvement of psoriasis with oral chondroitin sulfate: a serendipitous finding', *Dermatology* (2005).

(14) Brown, S.J., McLean, W.H., 'Current state of knowledge and future goals', *Journal of Investigative Dermatology* (2009).

(15) Kim, W.-J., et al, 'Relationship between serum IgA level and allergy/asthma', *The Korean Journal of Internal Medicine* (Korea, 2017).

(16) NHS Choices, 'The new guidelines on vitamin D – what you need to know', www.nhs.uk/news/food-and-diet/the-new-guidelines-on-vitamin-d-what-you-need-to-know/ (accessed on 21/06/2016).

2. THE LIVER

Anger and Frustration

Quietly efficient, the liver resides on the right-hand side of your body, in the upper quadrant, planning silently how to sweep up and filter the remnants of a good night out spent overindulging in alcohol and/ or eating a rich meal. This sophisticated glandular organ processes everything you eat and drink into energy and nutrients so that your body can use them to be the best possible you, but quite often we take the liver for granted and abuse it through overeating rich foods and drinking too much alcohol.

The liver is like a good friend who is (probably) always there, who listens and helps you without asking, who thinks ahead and does things for you that you didn't know you needed. But be warned! Even though the liver can regenerate itself, if you don't respect it through your nutritional choices, its capacity to perform this wizardry might run out.

The fresher the food you eat and the cleaner the water you drink, the better your liver performs (not to mention the more efficient your mind and body are at being the best version of you, physically and mentally). Good food and drink equals positive thinking and a strong physical body, whereas poor-quality food equals negative thinking and a weak physical body. The reason why you have bags under your eyes, spots on your jawline, dehydrated skin and bloodshot eyes all comes down to how well your liver filters and processes everything you eat and drink, so it makes sense that everything that goes into your mouth should be the best quality you can buy.

Facts:

- The liver weighs on average 1.3kg (2lb 14oz) – that's as much as a human brain.
- The liver is the only organ that can regenerate itself.
- 10 per cent of the liver is made up of fat.
- The liver is like a hoover that filters out alcohol, drugs and trans fats.
- The liver stores sugar for you to use as energy, like a battery.

A BIT MORE ANATOMY

The liver is often referred to as the grandfather of all organs because of the 500 tasks it performs daily, including fighting off infections, helping the blood to clot and neutralising toxins you take in from the air, the food you eat and drink and the drugs you take – both recreational and pharmaceutical.

The liver plays an important role in the body by regulating the flow of substances such as hormones, blood, bile and enzymes, to make sure they get to the right parts of the body at any given time, efficiently and effectively, so that your body works optimally. After the liver has broken down any harmful substances such as drugs, alcohol and chemicals, their byproducts are excreted into the blood or bile, are filtered out by the kidneys and leave the body in the form of urine or faeces. Your urine is a great way to test for health markers, and you can do this with a simple pH stick to test for protein, blood, nitrates, pH levels, ketones, bilirubin, liver stress and more. You can order these online very easily. You can also do these with your health professional and/or doctor.

The liver does its job of filtering and processing in the following three ways:

Carbohydrate metabolism: In the liver, excess glucose from the food you eat is converted to glycogen for storage in the liver before being used by the body as required. This ensures a constant energy supply in times of emergency. It is critical for the body to maintain concentrations of glucose in the blood within a narrow normal range of 70–99mg/dl, and these ranges are particularly important to the functioning of the liver.

Protein synthesis: The liver takes some protein, such as fish or beef, and breaks it down further into amino acids – the building blocks of protein. The liver converts essential amino acids (the ones that the body does not make) to non-essential amino acids (the ones the body does make). It also removes the nitrogen from the amino acids to form urea so it can be excreted via the urine.

Fat metabolism: Think about those times when you overeat, particularly carbohydrates. It may be because you are tired, hungover, bored or a bit low, and we all do it, so you are not alone. The problem is the body cannot utilise the excess carbohydrates you have eaten for energy, so your liver converts them into fatty acids and triglycerides, which are then exported and stored in your adipose tissue (fat tissue) to be used later.

When you overload the liver with toxins from smoke, drugs, environmental pollution, alcohol, processed food and such, it gets full or clogged up and the system stops filtering, and this is when problems occur. The good news is that reverse and regeneration are two major functions of the liver, so it's not too late to stop the damage if you change your ways. If you have liver cancer, for example, you can have nearly 70 per cent of your liver cut out and, provided the remaining 30 per cent is healthy, the liver will still function normally.

Although alcohol and processed food are the biggest enemies of the liver and also the most prevalent causes of liver disease, they are not the only ones. Liver disease is not always genetic; in fact, there are only a few conditions such as hemochromatosis, involving accumulation of iron in the body, and Wilson's disease, that are genetic to the liver – the rest are down to epigenetics and diet and lifestyle. Love your liver, love yourself.

Did you know?

For the Greeks, the liver was considered the seat of the emotions. They practised something called 'hepatoscopy', which involved sacrificing oxen or goats and examining their livers to determine whether their military campaigns would succeed or fail. The Greeks viewed the liver as the organ in closest contact with divinity.

ENERGIES OF THE LIVER

The meridian of the liver

The liver meridian begins with the big toe, ascends through the foot and the inner side of the leg and abdomen, and ends in the mid-thorax at the beginning point of the lung meridian. The liver meridian can affect the liver, the muscles, inner legs, groin, abdomen and ribs. If the liver meridian is out of balance you may experience liver problems, hepatitis, abdomen pain, vomiting, pancreatitis, jaundice, irregular menstruation and hernias.

Properties of the liver meridian

Force: Yin (female)

Chakra: Solar plexus – personal power, self-will

Organ body clock: 1–3am

Season: Spring

Colours: Green, blue-green

Fragrances: Sage, carnation and most sour aromas

Metaphysical lesson: Eliminating anger and proper expression of willpower

The emotions of the liver

Anger and frustration are the key emotions connected to the liver. Feelings of anger and frustration plague all of us at the best of times. We are all capable of flying off the handle, saying things we didn't mean or doing things that are out of character and having to apologise profusely for our actions. Sometimes anger stems from an underlying boredom or sometimes an underlying sense of fear or injustice disguised as anger. Our real emotions are lying just below the surface and we are too anxious, afraid, uncertain, scared or frustrated to let them out, or we don't know how to communicate our feelings efficiently, so instead we might resort to anger. Becoming aware that this is a pattern of behaviour and a trait of yours that is not benefiting you is the first step to making some changes.

THE FOUR BODIES OF THE LIVER

The spiritual body

The liver, on a spiritual level, is commonly associated with an inability to accept yourself or the circumstances you find yourself in.

When we are blissfully happy we don't need as much of a crutch to get us through the day – such as alcohol, drugs, bad food or any other addictions. When we are confused, stressed or in a state of resisting change these crutches block the situation so that you don't have to confront the issues but can simply hide behind them (see below).

Action: Start the day with a positive affirmation, such as I love and accept all the traits that make me who I am, the good, the bad and the ugly. I support them all with equal measure and intend to support my life by accepting myself.

The emotional body

The liver is very much an organ that holds the frustrations and manifestations of anger, as well as pain. It is also tied to feelings of envy, irritability, frustration, impatience and excessive ambition. On the positive side, the liver is also associated with healthier expressions of willpower, courage, confidence, contentment, satisfaction, enthusiasm, cooperation, acceptance and surrender.

The emotions you experience on a regular basis teach you about the health of your liver but equally bear in mind that how your liver functions can impact your emotions. If you spend more time at ease with who you are, what you are doing and where you are going, your liver will have an easier time of filtering and regulating, just as you are doing emotionally. Similarly, anger and resentment can undoubtedly damage the health of the liver.

Action: Find a quiet spot with no disruptions, and with a pencil and paper write down what or who is holding you back. What are you struggling to let go of? If you do not know, it is still important to write these thoughts down so that you are acknowledging that something needs to change for you to move on. If you like, throw the paper away afterwards so that no one will ever read it.

The nutritional body

Generally the foods that are good for the liver are vegetables, which are full of essential nutrients – such as broccoli, kale, spinach, cauliflower, garlic, horseradish and spring greens – and the darker green the better. You can juice these vegetables if you need to give your liver extra support, as that way the vitamins and nutrients will get into the bloodstream quicker and be transported around the body more efficiently. The liver also loves supplements such as milk thistle and chlorella, which again support the function of a stressed liver – especially one that has been exposed to toxins.

<u>Action</u>: Try sticking to regular or consistent mealtimes to support your liver, getting up and going to bed with the rise and fall of the sun. Make sure there is always something green on your plate that has come from Mother Nature!

The physical body

On a physical level, if you are experiencing digestive problems, circulation problems, red, dry or puffy eyes, retention of water or oedema, high cholesterol, high blood pressure, right shoulder pain, pain across the shoulder blades, lack of energy and an overall sense of not feeling well this could be a sign that your liver is in distress.

As its functions would indicate, the liver is intimately connected to a number of other organs, tissues and systems throughout the body, so there is always movement within each organ. The skin allows the body to sweat and by sweating we eliminate toxins. Sweat is best created by physical exercise and sometimes we can do too much of the high-intensity exercise like HIIT, running and boxing and we need to balance it with the working-in type of exercise, such as yoga or light jogging, that creates a parasympathetic response rather than a sympathetic response. The autonomic nervous system (ANS) regulates everything without asking or being prompted. It takes control of your blood pressure, heart rate, digestion, respiratory rate and sexual arousal and is controlled by a part of your brain called the hypothalamus. The hypothalamus is a bit like the Fat Controller in *Thomas the Tank Engine*, making sure everything works and runs efficiently! On either side of the ANS you have two branches: the parasympathetic nervous system (PNS) and the sympathetic nervous system (SNS). The PNS is responsible for rest and digestion while the SNS is the fight-or-flight side.

Find the right balance between working in and creating energy (parasympathetic) and working out and expending energy (sympathetic).

Action: Exercise increases heat and when done correctly can stimulate the liver. Exercise in the early morning or the early evening will support this organ the most. Try sticking to a routine when it comes to exercise, because adhering to a more predictable schedule can help keep your mind and body both cool and grounded. If you find yourself over-exercising, i.e. doing the same fast-paced high-intensity workout every day, try walking, hiking, swimming, cycling and yoga – all done with relaxed effort.

HOW TO LOOK AFTER YOUR LIVER

Your liver will look after you if you take regular exercise so that your body sweats, if you eat your green vegetables every day to help decrease the toxicity in your body, have more days without alcohol than with and find time to laugh and have fun.

Nutritional plan for a healthy liver

If you feel that you have been overdoing food or alcohol, partying to excess or simply feel like you need a bit of a health kick, here are some meals that you can incorporate into your day for variety and health.

Meals and snacks	Nutrition	Benefits
On waking in the morning	½ fresh organic lemon in warm filtered water	Highly detoxifying for the liver
First meal of the day	**Green vegetable juice:** Horseradish – 1 thumb-sized piece Garlic – ½ clove Broccoli – ½ head Spinach – 2 handfuls ½ cucumber 1 apple (optional) for taste	High in detoxification properties
Snack, if desired	**Apple and walnut crunch pot:** Chop a locally sourced apple into squares; add a handful of chopped walnuts and coat with 1 teaspoon of ground cinnamon. Toss in a frying pan with coconut oil for 2–3 minutes. Put in a glass jar so the flavours mix together before eating	The pectin in apples is great for digestion, and walnuts are full of omega 3
Second meal of the day	**Soft-boiled egg with rocket and cress salad:** Soft-boil 1 egg and sprinkle with paprika. Wash and tear equal amounts of rocket and watercress leaves. Drizzle with garlic-infused olive oil and lemon	Protein to avoid the afternoon slump with some bitter rocket leaves to aid digestion

Snack	Sea vegetable pot: Add 5 pieces of kombu and 25g (1oz) dried shiitake mushrooms to 1.2 litres (2 pints) of boiling water in a pan and let simmer for about 1 hour. Remove the sea vegetables and mushrooms, dice, and return to the pan. Add 1 teaspoon minced fresh ginger and simmer for 15 minutes. Stir in 1 tablespoon miso and garnish with chopped spring onions	Sea vegetables are full of iodine, manganese, vitamins C and B2 – so this is an all-round multivitamin meal
Third meal of the day	Dandelion and kimchi with sea trout: Bake 1 whole sea trout in an oven heated to 180°C/350°F gas 4 with salt, lemon and garlic to taste. Or in the summer months, barbecue the sea trout. Serve with dandelion and wet garlic leaves, washed, then tossed in olive oil and Celtic sea salt	Kimchi is great for the gut and sea trout is great for your skin, both are super-detoxing for the liver with dandelion leaves that help remove toxins and improve hydration
Bedtime snack	Dark berry pot: With a mortar and pestle, crush 2 tablespoons desiccated coconut and 1 teaspoon powdered or thumbnail-sized fresh ginger. Sprinkle over 1 handful of blueberries, raspberries and strawberries. Add a squeeze of lime	A bowl of antioxidants every day keeps the whole body happy!
	Cucumber basil and lemon water: Add ½ freshly squeezed lemon to some water with slices of ½ cucumber added. Crunch 4 basil leaves and add to the water	This water is extremely hydrating and refreshing

SIGNS THAT YOUR LIVER IS UNDER STRESS OR UNHAPPY

Dark circles under the eyes: Assuming you have not been up until 4am, dark shadows under the eyes can indicate you have a sub-optimal detoxification system, perhaps due to overconsumption of processed foods or alcohol.

Fatigue and malaise: We all get tired from time to time, but if you've felt consistently lethargic for a long time there could be a bigger issue at hand. A sluggish liver cannot filter the toxins and so creates imbalances elsewhere in the digestive, endocrine, and detoxification systems. Make sure you are eating foods that will keep it happy (see above), and book yourself a visit to a nutritionist.

Pain in the right shoulder: The body's communication system is made up of nerves and hormones. It is called the peripheral nervous system and it is a vast communication network, which transmits information between the brain, the spinal cord and the body. The nerves that feed the liver are known as T5-8 and feed the right shoulder. So if you are having consistent pain and no relief it may be time to look at the detoxification pathways and support your liver.

Loss of appetite: A loss of appetite can be the symptom of a congested liver, for which detoxification is recommended.

Blood pooling of the extremities (oedema) and abdomen (ascites): This is due to an increase of blood pressure in the portal vein (portal hypertension), which carries blood from the bowel and spleen to the liver and reduces the liver's ability to make a blood protein called albumin, therefore causing a pooling effect. If ascites is present you will look very bloated and your ankles may swell.

Jaundice: This is a condition where the body has excess bilirubin levels, which can present itself as having a yellow hue to the face and the whites of the eyes. It occurs when the bile stored in the liver fails to reach the duodenum of the small intestines, either because of a blockage, such as a gallstone, or a liver malfunction.

Steatorrhoea: This is otherwise known as floaty poos and is caused by undigested fat. The excretion of abnormal quantities of fat in the faeces can lead to a reduced absorption of fat by the intestine. Poo should sink and not float. If this carries on even after reducing the fat in your diet, you should have your stools tested for levels of fat by your GP. It may be a case of malabsorption of fat, and if so you need to support your digestive system and bile flow from the gallbladder.

Anger and jealousy: These two emotions can manifest when the liver becomes overwhelmed and struggles to detoxify.

Milk thistle for the liver

Milk thistle (*Silybum marianum*),[1] which has been used for 2,000 years, is an ancient herbal remedy for complaints of organs such as the liver, the gallbladder and the kidneys. Found within milk thistle is a substance called silymarin, which has antioxidant and anti-inflammatory properties, and this is thought to both protect and act as a remedy for ailments affecting these organs.

THE BIG DETOX!

The liver is a clever organ: it lets you know when it's unhappy (see page 67), and by now you hopefully have learnt a thing or two about your liver and what to do when you feel it needs some love. If you think yours does, you might consider a detox.

Everything starts with the mind, and detox is no exception. So while a detox is certainly something that is in vogue, it is not for everyone and its success is based on whether you have mentally committed to the process.

So what's the griff about detoxing? Often health professionals get very offended or uppity at the suggestion of a detox, because if you eat correctly for your metabolic type it's something that you shouldn't in theory have to do. Some people think that doing a juice cleanse is detoxing while some think giving up alcohol for a month has a similar effect. Some cut out cheese and meat, while some take milk thistle and B6 and carry on regardless. These 'detoxes' all work to some extent and contribute to what I refer to as damage control by improving the health and efficiency of your liver and accessory organs. I used to say to my ladies who would proudly tell me they were off to Turkey or Bali for a seven-day cleanse for a small fortune that they could go stay in my bathroom, for with its filtered water and filtered showers they would survive for seven days and come out feeling the same. My point is that while there are benefits to doing 'cleanses' like this, if you come back and resort to your old traits you've essentially wasted your time. Cleanses are a great kick-start for new healthy habits but they're not long-term solutions.

Most people give detoxing a shot in January when money is thin on the ground, we are tired from partying and the weather is cold – plus no one else is going out so it feels like a good time to take a break from the social scene. A month also seems a reasonable time to forego a few sins before picking up exactly where you left off, plus the sense of self-righteousness is gratification personified, smothering the need to continue this virtuous path of health any further.

But what is not always fully understood about the liver is that it is like a recycling chain. The liver detoxes and dumps everything it doesn't want into the colon. If the person has a ghetto gut (toxic gut), these liver metabolites will be reabsorbed by the colon and sent back to the liver, which in turn stores them and further congests the liver.

Cleanses and detoxes will only cause the recirculation back into the liver on a larger scale, which is otherwise known as enterohepatic circulation.

The point is that you detox every single second of the day, because that is how your body has been designed. If it didn't it would self-combust. Detoxification is part of the autonomic nervous system that just gets on with the job without instruction from you. The only thing you do is either make the process harder or easier depending on your diet and lifestyle choices.

The seven channels of elimination

Your body has seven channels of elimination: the liver, lymphatic system, kidneys, colon, lungs, skin and blood. The liver is much like a filter in the shower or a hoover; blood carries oxygen and nutrients to the cells and removes waste, and the lymphatic system is a network of tissues and organs that helps rid the body of toxins, waste and other unwanted materials. The kidneys filter the blood and essentially excrete waste as urine. The colon eliminates the waste as a bowel movement after all the nutrients have been absorbed. The lungs excrete carbon dioxide from the air you breathe and the blood helps this process, and waste products are taken in the blood to be filtered by the kidneys. The skin excretes salts, water and nitrogenous waste in the form of sweat or perspiration via the sweat glands.

So detoxification is about the optimal functioning of these seven channels and not just about cleansing with green juice and water for a week at a time.

Toxins

Toxins can come from two places: either inside the body (endogenous) or outside the body (exogenous). If exogenous toxins get into your body by being inhaled, ingested or absorbed into the bloodstream they can harm your cells. While we would not be able to live in a world free of exogenous toxins, we can try to reduce the amount that we are exposed to in our homes, workplaces, cars, food and environment; for example, MSG, recreational drugs, prescription drugs and beauty products.

Over time your gut can be a perfect hideout for toxins as the typical Western diet is rich in highly refined foods, fat, processed meats and table salt. If the cephalic response (see page 311) is not created – because of poor eating habits coupled with emotional stress – this can lead to an unhealthy balance of microorganisms in your gastrointestinal tract, a state known as intestinal symbiosis. Yeasts, fungi, bacteria and parasites all produce endogenous toxins known as endotoxins, which, once the infection has been irradiated, filter through the liver, which is why supporting the liver while on a gut health protocol is essential to ensure that more toxicity does not build up.

So with all these toxins entering the body, detoxification is an essential process by which blood must be cleansed, converting toxic metabolites to non-toxic metabolites to be carried out of the body. Most of the toxic chemicals that enter the body are fat-soluble, which means they dissolve in fatty or oily solutions and not in water, which makes it more difficult for the body to excrete them. Fat-soluble toxins also like to store themselves in fat tissue and cell membranes, and it is these tissues and membranes that can be stored for years, only released during exercise (which is why some people's sweat smells more than others'), or at times of stress or fasting. Since fatty tissue is mostly found in the brain and the endocrine system, (hormonal) dysfunction may set in in these areas, which may appear as infertility, breast soreness, adrenal exhaustion and early menopause. During this time you may experience symptoms of headaches, poor memory, stomach pain, nausea, fatigue, dizziness and palpitations, which are all common to detoxification.

In a study on the link between oestrogen and detoxification[2], oestrogen is principally synthesised in women by the ovaries and is detoxified and eliminated by the liver enzymes. So you can have a two-fold issue of excessive build-up of oestrogen in fat tissue and insufficient liver enzymes that are unable to process the oestrogen, leading to toxic overload. Diet plays a big role here, and a diet that is lacking the phase-two nutrients such as B vitamins, etc. will have difficulty metabolising the hormones and an increased risk of hormone-related problems such as fibroids, and even oestrogen-induced cancer.

In summary, the best way to keep all your channels of detoxification flowing and filtering efficiently is to make sure you're conscious of what you are putting into your body at all times.

ALCOHOL AND OTHER ADDICTIONS

The angry liver and its addictive nature

Addiction is more than a physiological illness, and thus its etiology lies deeper than the need for the addictive substance. Essentially this means that, for example, alcohol is not the problem for an alcoholic, food is not the reason why a person overeats, sugar is not the reason why someone is a sugar addict. The emotional body ties the substance to the emotion and creates the addiction and the dependency. Addiction is seen on the sympathetic side of the autonomic nervous system, creating a fight-or-flight response, an all-or-nothing situation, the feeling of being wired but tired, or living in the black or the white zone of addiction. If you find yourself suffering with addiction you could try acupuncture, which has been shown to increase the production of the body's natural opiates, which induce calm, quiet the fight-or-flight response and engender an overall sense of wellbeing.

Addiction can be seen as a result of an inability to adapt to the environment you find yourself in, for when you bond with the environment and people around you, you are content and happy. This then perpetuates, as we make more bonds when we are happy and feel safe. For some people making these bonds is challenging, perhaps because they have experienced a trauma, have a lack of confidence, or have been dealt a hard deck in life – such as growing up without a parent, or experiencing the death of a loved one at an early age. Trust can become an issue in these situations, which means bonds can be almost impossible to form, so instead these people seek a bond with something that gives instant gratification – and this is the main attraction in an addiction. Taking drugs and drinking alcohol every night, watching porn in secret, or racking up credit card bills on material things are not signs of happy people. Truly content, happy people have happy relationships that don't involve drinking a bottle of vodka night after night, because they choose to be present in their life.

Getting to the root of why you do what you do is paramount to getting rid of these addictions that ruin lives. You may find that addictive behaviours enable you to avoid confronting the real issues of why you have that behaviour in the first place. I have seen time and time again that when people with addictive natures start to address their diet and lifestyle, they lose their grip on the addiction. Removing the substance the person is addicted to may solve the problem in the short term, but if the emotional root cause is not dealt with the addiction will either return or rear its ugly head in some other manifestation.

One of my clients, Joanie, was best friends with vodka and fast food and suffered from bulimia and a lack of self-confidence. Her sessions with me would start with her being embarrassed to be seeing me again. She'd say, 'Oh Hannah, I can't believe I'm in the same place again, it's terrible, my gut is all over the place, my tummy hurts, I think I have throat cancer, my bowels are really smelly and I've been drinking. It's really bad, it is really bad, isn't it?'

Joanie had a habit of asking questions and then answering them herself, so much so that some sessions could be a long monologue of 'I hate me, I hate me', which I knew she loathed, but there just didn't seem a way out of this self-deprecating cycle. Yet sometimes we need to make the same mistake over and over, keep going around like a broken record until we become bored enough with our own story that we are inspired to do something to change it. Who or what was going to be the catalyst to induce change for Joanie, I pondered? Joanie had had a series of therapists who had gone some way to helping her, but I knew she was not addressing the root cause in these sessions because there was no change in her outlook on life or her reality in the time that I knew her. What did change was her environment; she changed jobs, she changed boyfriend, her financial situation changed, and from this creation of a new security her addictions started to have less of a grip on her.

Controlling her nutritional plan was the damage-control measure. If you are dealing with someone who drinks too much alcohol or who eats too much sugar or processed food, you would be a fool to think that you would be able to change them in one session. I use food and supplements to balance out the damage that the alcohol and poor food choices creates. Damage control is important because without these measures the health and vitality of the organs depletes and you get further away from health and the addictions get more em-bedded. If you can't decrease your intake or give up alcohol entirely, take a green supplement, vitamin B6, milk thistle or a liver support supplement to help the liver filter the excess alcohol. If you eat too much processed food, taking a probiotic, a digestive enzyme and an antioxidant will again help to break down this excess. Along the par-adigm of health, these are measures that will prevent an eventual pathology. We do not want to know that you do or do not have a disease, we want to know how close you are to that pathology so that you can take measures to get further away from that health state.

Joanie's answer was that she should give it all up; what she wanted to do was to not drink, but by taking the alcohol away with no other bond in place as a substitute, someone will only have a certain amount of self-discipline, willpower and strength before the vodka comes out of the freezer like a good faithful friend, always there in times of need. Unless you change the environment, you have changed nothing. Similar is true of relationship break-ups; often people go to the other side of the world to find themselves, only to find a different scenery. I say going to a new coffee shop would be cheaper, and probably just as effective!

So why do so many people find it so hard to give up all the bad stuff? Why are patterns so hard to change for some but not for others? For healthy relationships to exist with food, people, family, work, etc. there must be a few things in place first, such as accountability, safety, honesty, support, cooperation and trust.

Am I a functioning alcoholic?

Most people would say no when asked this question, but as I am in a more advantaged place of seeing the habits and traits of what people do on a daily basis, in most cases I'd say they are functioning alcoholics!

I see food diaries and hear first-hand of 70-year-old men and women who drink champagne with lunch and before dinner every day, which minimally is 14 units a week. Some would say how civilised, some would not! There are also 40-year-olds who drink one or two glasses of wine every evening to wind down from stressful, unenjoyable jobs and fast-paced lifestyles, and there are the bingers who spend weekends fuelled by cocktails of alcohol and drugs.

The image of a drunk old man on the street is one that most people associate with being an alcoholic, but the truth is alcoholics just as often have well-paid jobs, families and homes, and spotting these people is slightly harder. Regular drinkers may slip into alcoholism; a drink at lunchtime can quickly spiral into the need for a drink every lunchtime and it can become a drug you have to feed yourself in order to experience the same feeling and sensation of confidence or freedom. The downward spiral that occurs before people seek help is unfortunately one that can happen with great ease and speed.

For some, alcohol has far-reaching problems; the drinking doesn't just stop at the end of the night. Alcohol can begin to affect relationships, financial situations, social activities, health and an individual's future. The reasons why some people become dependent on alcohol and why some are more susceptible than others to misuse the substance have many variables and is a well-researched and vast subject. For the best possible you, it is important to be able to recognise the health symptoms associated with the misuse of alcohol so that you can identify whether or not you need to take some action, and, if so, how you can help to support your health and that of your liver, which takes the brunt of this overconsumption.

In my practice the big question I hear, especially among middle-aged men and women, is: 'Are you going to tell me to stop drinking alcohol, and are you going to tell me to stop drinking coffee?' I say no, why would I do that? If I take away your treat, your 'vice', your crutch, with no support you'll probably last about two days before falling harder than you did before. That's setting someone up for failure, which is what most wellness plans do. Instead, I say to them, I want you to tell me that you no longer wake up in the morning looking forward to that coffee to drag you out of bed, or that you have swapped two nights with Chardonnay for two nights with a class pass at your local fitness studio. It is an educational process, one of trial and error, and my job, I tell them, is for you to extract all my knowledge so that you start to recognise the signs and symptoms of an out-of-balance mind and body so that you can be your own doctor.

Kicking the habit is about changing the pathways to create a different outcome. Sometimes we have to make mistakes time and time again before we accept that what we are doing simply isn't making us happy. This is not only true with alcohol but with anything that can be called an addictive trait, anything that we find hard to let go of and recognise as no longer serving us.

Once you embrace the failure-to-success ratio you are well on your way to achieving your own success or helping other people to achieve theirs. The most successful among us in any field are those who have failed the most; it is part of life's journey and education and should be embraced and not feared. Failing is predictive of a highly intuitive and motivated individual who will ultimately succeed in any field. Welcome failure as hard work, endurance of character and perseverance of the dream, as it is the only predictor of success in life.

The hangover plan!

Alcohol, as we know, is toxic to your liver, and it is your liver that has to process alcohol, so the more you drink, the more work your liver has to do and the more painful the hangover will be in the morning.

If you drink too much on occasion, this is my advice for making the healing process the most efficient and effective.

Working out your alcohol consumption

First, you need to know how long alcohol stays in your system. Three units (a large 250ml (9fl oz) glass of wine at 12 per cent) will take three hours to metabolise. Beer can be anywhere from 2.3–3.4 units, depending on the strength of the beer, and on average takes two hours to metabolise. Being able to add up units is a really beneficial skill to have, especially if you have to work the next day or you can't afford to be confined to the sofa or, more importantly, you want to have the healthiest liver and detoxification system possible.

If you drink a large glass of wine – that's three units for wine at around 12–13 per cent alcohol – your body will take about three hours to break down the alcohol. So if you can (honestly) easily drink a bottle of white wine by yourself over the course of the evening and you start drinking at 7.30pm, finishing the bottle by 9.30pm, and the wine is 12 per cent alcohol, that's nine units you've drunk. In that case, the alcohol will be clear at 5.30am, 10 hours later, as the first unit takes two hours to break down. So you can see how easy it is to be over the drink-driving limit in the morning, but also why you feel groggy until lunchtime. Other variables do need to be taken into consideration and timings may differ, but it is always better to over-evaluate than under-evaluate the time taken for alcohol to be cleared from the blood. Other considerations will be body fat, size, age, height-to-weight ratio and speed of consumption.

The pretox

It's all about damage control; the less you drink, the less of this you will have to do (although alcohol does affect each of us to varying degrees). Before you go out for a night that may involve drinking, take some supplements to reduce the effects of the alcohol in the morning; whichever of the following you take, it is important to find plant-based supplements, as they are more effective and non-toxic on the liver.

NAC: Take 200mg 30 minutes before you have your first drink to lessen the effects of alcohol. NAC is a form of the amino acid cysteine; it is known to help increase glutathione and reduce the acetaldehyde toxicity that causes many hangover symptoms.[3]

B6: Deficiencies of B6 are found in people who have liver disease.[4] It is the most underrated vitamin, which helps the body do almost everything.[5] B6 is your best friend, and it can be found in bananas, avocados, broccoli (in higher amounts in frozen broccoli than raw), cauliflower and almonds. Vitamin B6 is unstable to alkaline conditions, light, oxygen and high temperatures, so much of the B6 originally present in foods can be lost in processing, such as prolonged or high heating, canning and pressure cooking, milling of grains into refined flour, sterilisation and freezing (although this doesn't apply to all foods, as stated above with broccoli).

Magnesium: One of the most abundant minerals in the body and, for many, this is also the most depleted because of modern lifestyles and city living. Magnesium deficiency is primarily caused by the agribusiness farming practices that have stripped our soils of vital minerals needed for health. It is becoming clear that a diet high in magnesium, and therefore fruits and vegetables, is essential. Several studies have revealed magnesium deficiency in clients with liver cirrhosis, who show considerably reduced muscle strength and muscle Mg.[6] Magnesium may have a role in the neuromuscular and neuropsychiatric manifestations of chronic liver disease (hepatic encephalopathy and muscle cramps).

Milk thistle[7]: The liver can, of course, function without milk thistle, but it is significantly less under strain when it is aided by this well-known herb. Incorporate milk thistle into your diet and you can maintain optimum liver health in combination with a healthy diet and lifestyle.

Vitamin C: In some studies vitamin C has been proven to be better as a protective mechanism than milk thistle. Again, this is another vitamin that is depleted when you drink alcohol, so make sure you take it in a supplement form as well as include it in your diet plan.

The hangover detox

Keep it light, keep it clean and keep it green! This is your hangover plan.

Time	Nutrition	Active ingredient
Before you get into bed	Probiotic, 0.5 litre (1 pint) of water, 2 x chlorella tablets and 1 x vitamin C	Good bacteria – for gut health; vitamin C – antioxidant; chlorella – helps drag the toxins out from the night
Upon waking	0.5 litre (1 pint) of water with ½ lemon with the rind on, squeezed 1 glass of coconut water	Hydration – for potassium levels and kidney support

10 hours after your last drink **Breaking the fast!**	Green juice – ½ avocado, ½ banana, 1 tablespoon nut butter and 1 tablespoon olive oil, 250ml (9fl oz) coconut water, 1 tablespoon green powder and 1 teaspoon raw honey	Electrolytes – to rehydrate; avocado, nut butter, olive oil – good fats; honey – antibacterial
30–60 minutes after breakfast	2 x innate plant-based digestive enzymes with 100ml water	Plant-based enzymes for digestion and absorption
20 minutes later	Turmeric and cayenne peppered eggs with steamed Tenderstem broccoli	Plant-based enzymes for digestion and absorption
Activity	Get some fresh air and go for a walk	To clear the mind and wake up the muscles
Lunch	**If you need some comfort food:** Grilled chicken thighs with buckwheat noodles, spinach, red onion and dairy-free pesto **If you don't need comfort food:** A bowl of chicken bone broth – see page 81; or spiralised courgettes with salmon flakes and basil-infused olive oil	Cysteine for healing (see below)
Throughout the afternoon	**Make a pot of tea:** Raw honey and ginseng root Lemon and ginger Green tea Lemon leaves	Digestion

Dinner	**Mum's chicken soup:** Chicken stock or broth with diced carrots, celery, cider apple vinegar, tomatoes and garden herbs	Inflammation

Cysteine severely reduces the effects of a hangover as it creates antioxidants in the body. Cysteine is a natural amino acid found in chicken and other meats which can thin the mucus in your lungs and make it less sticky and so easier for you to propel. Perfect after a hangover, to expel those wastes. (Cysteine has also been proven to play a role in reducing the symptoms of asthma.)

By adding spices to a chicken broth the watery fluids in your lungs will help thin down the respiratory mucus, also making it easier to expel. Stock contains minerals in a form that makes it easy for the body to absorb; it contains the broken-down cartilage and tendons that you find in the supplements called glucosamine. It is cheaper to drink medicinal broth than buy a supplement, which also saves you money and will relieve your joint pain. Glucosamine is the supplement you take when you want to support the pain in your body and reduce inflammation, or if you have arthritis. Glutathione is made by cysteine and is a bit like a magnet – it attracts all the bad stuff and expels it. It is the master amino acid for this reason.

How to make bone broth
- 1.5kg (3lb 5oz) grass-fed or organic bones
- 2 chicken feet for extra gelatin (optional), add with bones
- 3 tablespoon organic apple cider vinegar
- 1 white onion, chopped
- 2 carrots, chopped
- 2 celery sticks, chopped
- 1 tablespoon sea salt

- 1 teaspoon black peppercorns
- 1 teaspoon juniper berries
- 3 garlic cloves
- 1 bunch of parsley

Equipment you will need:
- Slow cooker or large stockpot
- Strainer to remove the pieces when finished
- Pestle and mortar for the juniper berries

1   Preheat the oven to 180°C/350°F gas 4. To improve the flavour of the bones, first place them in a roasting pan and roast for 30 minutes.

2   Remove the bones from the oven and place them in a large pot or slow cooker. Pour (filtered) water over the bones and add the cider vinegar – the acid helps make the nutrients in the bones more available. Let sit for 20–30 minutes in the cool water.

3   Add the onion and vegetables to the pot or slow cooker, followed by the sea salt, black pepper and juniper berries, crushed using the pestle and mortar.

4   Simmer the bones and vegetables for 8–10 hours over a low heat. Check on it from time to time – if a residue forms on the surface, remove this with a slotted spoon. Grass-fed and healthy animals will produce much less of this than conventional animals.

7   Add the garlic and parsley during the last 30 minutes of cooking.

8   Once finished cooking, let the broth cool slightly, then strain using a fine metal strainer to remove all the bits of bone and vegetable.

9   Once it has cooled you can drink it immediately, or transfer it to a large glass jar and store it in the fridge for up to 5 days, or freeze for later use.

Other herbs/supplements to support a hangover
Milk thistle: This is just as useful after drinking as it is before. Milk thistle is able to assist your liver, which is designed to detoxify the

chemicals that enter the body from the environment and the food we eat, in combination with a healthy diet and lifestyle.

Dandelion: The bitterness of this leaf supports liver function because bitters aid digestion, while the potassium contained within it helps to flush impurities out of the body via the kidneys and urine.

Celery seed: Often used as a diuretic, it also helps flush out toxins.

Cayenne pepper: Stimulates your circulatory system, including boosting your lymphatic system, digestive systems and rhythms. The heat from the pepper helps your gastric juices to flow, increasing your body's ability to metabolise food and toxins.

Green tea: Research has now proven that drinking green tea is beneficial in reducing inflammation in the body and providing a super-dose of antioxidants.[8]

Other ways to support a hangover

Exercise: It is always good to get some fresh air into the lungs and change the scenery from being inside the house, so go for a walk around the block, take the dog for a stroll or perhaps even a light jog. Exercising the day after a heavy night is never a bad thing as it will help you sweat the toxins out of the skin. The aim is to get rid of these toxins, which will not only be alcohol, but all sorts of other extras that creep in – the sugar from the alcohol encourages you to eat food on the way home from a night out.

Be kind to yourself: You can sometimes have a feeling of paranoia when you wake up the morning after a night out. Did you behave badly, did you send an inappropriate text or leave a brave voicemail? Were you Mr or Mrs Inappropriate at the event? The most important thing to remember is that these feelings are fleeting and they will go, and you will feel emotionally strong again when you put your hangover plan into place. Keep doing what you need to do to feel better and don't spend the day eating sugary treats as this will fuel your anxiety and make matters worse. Refer to the plan on pages 79–80 instead.

PATHOLOGIES OF THE LIVER

If the liver suffers a trauma it can and does heal and regenerate. If the liver suffers persistent traumas this can lead to fibrosis of the liver, then cirrhosis of the liver, resulting in liver failure. The main causes of liver trauma are excessive intake of alcohol or processed or fatty foods. It is important to recognise these issues and, more importantly, to see if you recognise them in you. Liver disease is on the rise in the UK according to the BMJ[9], more than any other chronic condition. It goes on to say that alcohol and obesity are to blame, alcohol consumption has doubled per person in the last half-century and one in four adults are considered to be obese. Both preventable causes!

Alcoholic hepatitis

This is an inflammation of the liver and is usually due to an excessive intake of alcohol. It is also associated with a fatty liver, an early stage of alcoholic liver disease, and may contribute to the progression of fibrosis leading to cirrhosis.

What alcoholic hepatitis may look and feel like
- **Jaundice:** See page 89.
- **Ascites:** Accumulation of fluid in the peritoneum in the abdominal cavity. This can be caused by a constrictive pericarditis (a thickened, fibrotic pericardium that restricts heart expansion). You may not have any symptoms (asymptomatic), or you may experience abdominal pain and bloating and a shortness of breath.
- **Fatigue and hepatic encephalopathy:** This is a brain dysfunction due to liver failure. Mild cases are self-limiting, but severe cases have a

high risk of death. Severe cases may be treated with glucocorticoids (a steroid hormone that reduces inflammation).

Non-alcoholic fatty liver disease (NAFLD)

If it's not alcohol that is going to cause liver disease, it will be fatty food. In fact, fatty food is now the leader in the causes of liver disease, a condition that is extremely prevalent in children. In some cases NAFLD can develop into non-alcoholic steatohepatitis (NASH), which is where the liver cells are filled with more fat than they can handle, causing inflammation of the liver. ('Steato' means fat, and 'hepatitis' means inflammation of the liver.) You can prevent or cure fatty liver disease through reversing lipotoxicity and insulin resistance via diet and lifestyle intervention.

Who develops NAFLD?

NAFLD is the most common persistent chronic liver disorder in Western countries; it is thought to occur in about one in five adults in the UK and in up to four in five adults who are obese. (However, most of these people have 'simple fatty liver' and not the more serious types of NAFLD.) It is commonly associated with insulin resistance, obesity, dyslipidaemia, type 2 diabetes and cardiovascular disease. Its pathogenesis is complex and so is its diagnosis, which can only be made using a biopsy. Health screening is vital to establish potential causes such as medication and alcoholism.

NAFLD is increasing not only in the adult population but amongst children too. It's now estimated that NAFLD will be the leading cause of all liver pathologies in western countries in the next 10 years[10]. It's sad to see that in western countries where we have everything we need and want at a fingertip that our food supply is poisoning us slowly with dramatic effect. Insulin resistance and obesity (the main causes of NAFLD) are caused by foods that are not from mother nature but created in factories and are therefore putting untold amounts of stress on the body. The great news is that an early diagnosis enables the body to heal itself, which you can do simply with clean food, water, exercise and deep sleep.

What are some of the symptoms associated with NAFLD and what might it look or feel like to you?

Most people with simple fatty liver or NASH have no symptoms; however, some people have a persistent nagging pain in the upper right part of the tummy (abdomen) over an enlarged liver, which is the key indicator of an imbalanced liver.

Enlarged breasts in men (gynaecomastia): This is caused by a hormone imbalance between testosterone and oestrogen. Males and females have both these hormones; oestrogen makes breast tissue grow and testosterone has inhibitory effects, i.e. it prevents oestrogen growing breast tissue.

Red palms (Palmar erythema): Red palms are a common indicator of alcoholism and pathologies of the liver.

Jaundice: See page 89.

Blood in stools: In the later stages of cirrhosis you may vomit blood or have tarry, black stools. This is because blood can't flow through the liver properly, which causes an increase in blood pressure in the vein that carries blood from the gut to the liver (portal vein). The increase in blood pressure forces blood through smaller, fragile vessels that line your stomach and gullet (varices). These can burst under high blood pressure, leading to internal bleeding which is visible in vomit and your stools.

Fluid retention (ascites): Swelling in your tummy (abdomen) caused by a build-up of fluid known as ascites – severe cases can make you look heavily pregnant.

Itchy skin (pruritus): This is a common symptom, but it does not always occur. It is sometimes severe and distressing and makes the whole skin feel itchy. The cause of the itch is not always clear – it may be due to a chemical from the bile, which builds up in the bloodstream.

Obesity: Most people with NAFLD are obese or overweight; if this is you, it is worth getting some liver function tests.

Diabetes: Having type 2 diabetes increases the chances of developing NAFLD, but there is no connection between this condition and type 1 diabetes.

Hyperlipidaemia: If you have high levels of cholesterol and/or triglycerides in your blood you have a higher risk of developing NAFLD.

What you should be eating to prevent and reverse fatty liver disease
Changing your diet to incorporate and focus on the foods listed below will reduce the amount of fat accumulating in the liver, improve insulin function, make weight loss a lot easier and help reverse NAFLD.

Foods to include in every meal, every day	How much?	Why?
Raw plant food, especially vegetables that are in season and organic. Fruits are good but contain a high amount of sugar, so eat more vegetables than fruit if you are trying to lose weight	You can eat an unlimited amount of vegetables but a sensible guideline would be to have two different varieties of vegetable in season with every main meal and limit fruit to 2–4 pieces a day. Eat them raw if you do not have digestive problems; steamed are easier to digest if you do	Vegetables are full of nutrients and vitamins that are essential for health and prevent deficiencies

All meat, poultry and fish, as well as eggs, legumes or a quality protein powder	Proteins make you feel satisfied, so having them in some form at every meal will prevent you craving more carbohydrates or overeating	Lean organic protein is the building block for your muscles; muscles house all your internal organs and keep them working
Cooked vegetables that grow underground, such as roasted spicy sweet potatoes or squash	One portion with either lunch or dinner	These make up for the fact that you are not eating bread and pasta, biscuits and sugary desserts as they are complex carbohydrates
Choose from the following snacks, 1–2 per day		
Raw nuts and seeds with or without fruit	One handful of nuts/ seeds and one piece of fruit	The good fats from the nuts will keep you satisfied and the sweetness from the fruit will make you happy. A perfect combination
Avocado/hummus/ bean dips with raw vegetable sticks	1 tablespoon per day	A good snack or starter, to keep you nutritionally satisfied
Cold-pressed vegetable juice	One per day, max 250ml (9fl oz)	Vegetables in liquid form get the nutrients transported around the body as quickly and efficiently as possible
Protein smoothie with coconut or almond milk and fresh berries	One per day, 330ml (11fl oz)	Perfect if your job is more physically active. Liquid with protein and fat stays in the stomach longer, keeping you satisfied for longer, too

Listen to your body and follow your natural instincts when it comes to the amount of food you need to eat to feel satisfied and happy. It is not how much you eat that counts, it is what you are eating that is so important for your liver and insulin levels.

What else you can do to prevent getting a fatty liver

Move more: The benefits of exercise are endless and there is no exception when you have NAFLD. It is important for every system in the body to move and for the body to sweat, which helps excrete toxins and waste. Exercise reduces hepatic inflammation, lowers elevated liver enzyme levels and decreases insulin resistance, which helps maintain blood sugar levels to prevent diabetes and obesity. If you are new to exercise, take it slowly at first, but try to build up to a sweat. Walking 10,000 steps a day is a good place to start, then aim to build it up until you are running 5 km (3 miles). Listen to your body, but try to do some physical exercise for 30 minutes five days a week.

Emotionally engage: If you can connect the way you move and the way you feel, you start to become emotionally intelligent and aware of how food makes you feel. Start to associate the positive feelings with a clean and healthy diet and lifestyle choices, then you will begin to associate previous feelings of anger, frustration and anxiety with the way you used to eat – we are more likely to eat badly when we are feeling low. Try keeping a mood and food diary. In one column list your mood and in the other the foods that you are eating, to give you a bespoke plan of which make you happy and which make you sad.

Jaundice

Although not a disease, jaundice is a sign of underlying disease. The word jaundice comes from the French word *jaune*, meaning yellow. Jaundice occurs when the bile pigment, bilirubin, builds up to an abnormally high level in the blood and fails to reach the duodenum, either because of a blockage, such as a gallstone, or liver malfunction. This condition is also referred to as icterus, the yellow staining of the skin and sclera (whites of the eyes). Bilirubin is a yellowish-brown product that is found in bile and is produced when the liver breaks down red blood cells. It is excreted in urine and bile and when elevated may cause disease states. Jaundice may also be caused by too many red blood cells dying at once or too much bilirubin being present in the liver at one time. A correct and timely diagnosis of these conditions is essential for finding a suitable treatment plan.

Jaundice is quite common in newborns, particularly 48 to 72 hours after birth. This condition is thankfully benign, disappearing within two weeks. But there is a rare, chronic type of jaundice caused by an increase in the destruction of red blood cells. A good test to see if the jaundice is leaving the body is to press down on the newborn's nose – on release of pressure there should be no sign of a yellow tone to the skin.

What jaundice might look or feel like to you
Dark urine: Often the first urination of the day is darker in colour; however, if the urine is consistently dark in colour throughout the day you may want to investigate further, especially if you think you drink enough water.

Yellow glow to skin: Often people do have a yellow look to them, which can be mistaken for an overdose of beta carotene and can have the same effect. You get beta carotene from carrots, which converts to vitamin A, which we need for good vision. However, jaundice is not desirable, so you need to be able to spot the difference.

Pale stools: These signify a problem with the drainage of your biliary system, which is comprised of your gallbladder, liver and pancreas. The pale colour comes from the bile salts that are released from your liver.

Certain medicines: Drugs like acetaminophen (paracetamol), penicillin, birth-control pills and steroids have been linked to liver disease.

How to test for jaundice
In the early stages treatment might be a case of rapidly changing your

lifestyle habits. If you have had some liver tests, such as AST and ALT, you would be able to ascertain if you have jaundice. Non-invasive methods exist to find the cause of jaundice, such as an ultrasound or computed tomography and laboratory testing.

Minimally invasive techniques include cholangiography (which creates an image of bile ducts), endoscopic retrograde cholangiopancreatography (ERCP) and percutaneous transhepatic cholangiography (injecting an image-enhancing dye directly into the liver).

Other diseases underlying jaundice can include cirrhosis, thalassaemia, hepatitis A and cholestasis; these are either inherited or are auto-immune disorders, so they cannot be prevented. If you have acute viral hepatitis, jaundice will go away on its own as the liver begins to heal. If a blocked bile duct is to blame, your doctor may suggest surgery to open it.

So if you feel like your body needs a break or that you have been overdoing it recently, it is probably time to take some me-time and to put together a spring-clean programme for your body.

The niacin flush: a spring-clean for your liver

This will get you moving!

What you need:
- A sauna
- Niacin – B3
- Activated charcoal tablets

Niacin is one of the B vitamins that induces a strong flushing reaction. Look for the 100mg tablets and take 50mg per 20kg (44 lb) of body weight; wait for roughly 20 minutes and then jump on the cross trainer or do some bodyweight exercises until you break sweat and stimulate circulation, then follow up with a hot sauna. Stay in the sauna for as long as you can cope with, and drink water if you need to. It is not about staying in the sauna for as long as you can, though, so take as many breaks as you need; it is about getting your body to sweat. The niacin forces your body to sweat and flush out toxins and can induce a tingling feeling or itchiness. The idea is that the niacin and the sweating stimulate fat breakdown because lots of chemicals are stored in fat.

Have a shower set to a regular body temperature and take some time to sit down and rest. You can then have a glass of water with some charcoal tablets or chlorella tablets which will help pull out more toxicity, which is being eliminated through the gastrointestinal tract.

This flush can be used as part of any cleansing regime.

TOP 10 TIPS FOR A HEALTHY LIVER

1. **Drink more water:** *The Body's Many Cries for Water* by F. Batmanghelidj[11] is not just a recommended read, it's an essential read, and if you are one of the copious water haters out there it needs to be on your wish list. F. Batmanghelidj's 25-year study covers the most underrated health cure for many ills. If you were depressed, you'll be happy; if you were dehydrated, you'll be hydrated; if you were in pain, you'll be out of pain and if you were overweight you'll get back into balance – and all you have to do is drink more water. Not liking water is otherwise known as unintentional chronic dehydration (UCD) and is self-regulated!

2. **Eat beetroot:** Not only because it's the coolest colour of all the vegetables but when you add ginger to a beetroot juice something quite magical happens – add mint and you are in heaven, then add a shot of apple and you are quite simply in an oasis of health. On a serious note, it's your liver's best friend because of the betacyanin responsible for the vibrant colour, but it also speeds up something called phase two detoxification – a process that takes the nasties out of your body. So get beet juicing!

3. **Throw lemons over everything:** Squeeze, juice, drink, grate, grind

– just make sure there are lemons in your life. A natural liver and gall-bladder cleanser as well as a great source of vitamin C, put lemons in water in the morning, in your fruit salad to slow down oxidation at lunch, in your tea in the afternoon and in your honey and lemon drink at night.

4. **Milk thistle:** Milk thistle assists your liver, which is designed to detoxify the chemicals that enter the body from the environment and the food we eat. Milk thistle protects the liver by absorbing a lot of chemicals and toxins that would otherwise be dangerous. Incorporate this into your diet and you can maintain optimum liver health when combined with a healthy diet and lifestyle.

5. **Discover rainbow chard:** Chard is a little-known treasure in the world of vegetables and a very close relative of beetroot. Betacyanin is the compound giving colour to the veins of the leaves and speeding up chemical functions within the liver, which break down toxic matter and remove it from the body. This is a process involved in phase two liver detoxification.

6. **Eat artichokes:** This vegetable is almost a completely different-looking plant when it is pre-packaged in supermarkets to the one that is picked in its natural habitat. It is one of the most potent liver cleansers, which is why you will find it in most liver support supplements. The caffeoylquinic acid in it helps stimulate the bile flow from the liver to the gallbladder. So as it removes the toxins from your liver you also see your skin brighten up.

7. **Spring-clean your house:** The liver is said to be the organ that efficiently holds feelings of anger and frustration. So not only do we need to look after our diet for an efficiently working liver, we must also clear out our lives of all the material things we do not need, of the relationships that no longer serve us, and of the negative thoughts and emotions that plateau us and stump our progress. Doing so will make you feel lighter and more in charge of your life.

8. **Remove energy robbers:** Write a list of all the things and all the people

in your life who perhaps take more than they give. It is good to be able to reflect on exactly where you are expending your energy. Sometimes these energy robbers become common practice, which doesn't mean to say they are the norm. If you are giving out more than you are getting back, you need to address the imbalance.

9. **Fast one day a week:** We regularly overload our digestive system and therefore the liver too, as it has to filter the overeating and overdrinking. Mondays are a good day to drink more water, vegetable juices and green tea, particularly after a weekend of indulgence.

10. **Forgive yourself:** There is one life that we know of and one body that you inhabit, so beating yourself up about things you have done or have had no control over in the past is fruitless. Accept your dark side as much as you like all the qualities of your light side – it is the dark traits that make you who you are and without them you would not be you – then move on. One body, one chance.

Footnotes

(1) Marciano, M., Vizniak, N., 'Botanical Medicine: Herbs, nutrition, hormones & medications', Professional Health Systems Inc. (Canada, 2018).

(2) Hall, D., 'Nutritional Influences on Estrogen Metabolism', *Applied Nutritional Science Reports* (2001).

(3) Khoshbaten, M. et al, 'N-Acetylcysteine Improves Liver Function in Clients with Non-Alcoholic Fatty Liver Disease', *Hepatitis Monthly* (Tehran, 2010).

(4) Labadarios, D. et al, 'Vitamin B6 deficiency in chronic liver disease – evidence for increased degradation of pyridoxal-5'-phosphate', *Gut* (BMA London, 1977).

(5) Leevy, C.M. et al, 'Complex vitamins in liver disease of the alcoholic', *American Journal of Clinical Nutrition* (Maryland, 1965).

(6) 'Magnesium in liver cirrhosis', www.ClinicalTrials.gov (accessed on 10/01/2016).

(7) Jacobs, B.P. et al, 'Milk thistle for the treatment of liver disease: A systematic review and meta-analysis', *American Journal of Medicine* (Arizona, 2002).

(8) Lambert, J., Elias, R., 'The antioxidant and pro-oxidant activities of green tea polyphenols: A role in cancer prevention', *Archives of Biochemistry and Biophysics* (San Diego, 2010).

(9) Ratib, S., West, J., Fleming, K.M., 'Liver cirrhosis in England – an observational study: are we measuring its burden occurrence correctly?' *BMJ Open* (London, 2017).

10) Temple, Jonathan L., et al, 'A Guide to Non-Alcoholic Fatty Liver Diseases in Childhood and Adolescence, *International Journal of Molecular Sciences* (Basel, 2016).

(11) Batmanghelidj, F., *The Body's Many Cries for Water* (Tagman Press, 2000).

3. THE GALLBLADDER

Envy and Jealousy

Your gallbladder is a little pear-shaped organ roughly 4 centimetres (1½ inches) in length which can be found in the upper right quadrant of the abdomen. Its job is to hold bile, made in the liver, and break down fat. It is one of the smallest organs in the body and unfortunately it has been marked as one that you can live without, which explains why not much attention is paid to it; that is, until it goes wrong and starts causing chronic pain, at which point instant action may be required.

The gallbladder has one of the most important and tasty jobs in the body: it gets to break down fat! Fat is the tastiest of all macronutrients by far and leaves us feeling satisfied. When we take fat out of the meal we become less satisfied and crave sugar. Sometimes when we are trying to lose weight we cut out fat but this tactic relies on having willpower of steel as you battle through the plain and uninspired grilled salmon salads and plates of boiled chicken and broccoli. With every meal, breaking point gets closer until you can bear it no longer and you unlock the biscuit tin, or take the chains off the fridge and dive into those good old-fashioned carbohydrates, providing you with instant gratification. The problem with this, however, is that if you take away the fat then it's only a matter of time before the carb cravings start, and that is counterproductive.

Don't be scared of fat – your gallbladder breaks it down efficiently and uses it for energy. Just make sure you eat the right fats (see page 110).

So what is the role of the gallbladder? It receives bile from the liver, ready for when the small intestines need it during digestion. When you eat food, the cells of the intestines produce a hormone called cholecystokinin, which causes the gallbladder to contract and release the bile into the small intestines via the common bile duct. In a healthy gallbladder this process happens painlessly; however, when the gallbladder stops working properly or the bile ducts are blocked, this can cause a lot of pain and discomfort.

If you don't make time to be well now you'll have to take time later to be sick. Learn what the parts of your body do and how to look after them before you have to discover how hard it is to live without them.

On a psycho-emotional level, it is good to remember that the gallbladder stores daily stress.

Facts:

- The gallbladder stores bile, it does not make it. If you don't have a gallbladder you have nowhere to store bile.
- It is the organ most frequently removed from the body, in a surgery known as a cholecystectomy.
- A low-fat diet increases the formation of gallstones.

A BIT MORE ANATOMY

The gallbladder is part of the human biliary system, which means it is responsible for the storage, production and transportation of bile. It acts as a reservoir for bile flowing through the hepatic ducts from the liver into the gallbladder and from there to the duodenum, which is the first part of the small bowel, and then on to emulsify fats and to excrete some products such as bilirubin and cholesterol. Bilirubin is a waste product that is eliminated from the body by being secreted through bile and expelled in faeces, but it also works to maintain a healthy microorganism balance.

The importance of bile

Bile is a lubricant that emulsifies fat, cholesterol and the fat-soluble vitamins A, D, E and K that come into the body in your food, breaking them down into smaller particles. This creates a larger surface area for lipase (fat enzymes) to act on during digestion. An insufficiency of bile makes it hard for your body to break down fats.

Foods that help stimulate bile production are called cholagogues. Often you can find these in a combination supplementation form but to get them into your diet from food sources, try radish, turnip greens, mustard greens, chicory, dandelion and artichokes. Herbs that are cholagogues include wormwood, blue flag and fringe tree. So the good news is that you can eat foods that help bile products and fat emulsification, thereby looking after your gallbladder naturally.

The best way to look after your gallbladder is to support your small intestine by eating good fats (we'll come back to this later) such as avocado or ghee. This causes the hormones of the digestive tract to stimulate and secrete cholecystokinin (CCK) and secretin – the hormone kings of appetite and digestion – from the duodenum and jejunum of the small intestines.

It also persuades enzymes and liquids from the pancreas to further assist in the breakdown of fats, carbohydrates and proteins. Secretin, a digestive hormone, is also secreted when partially broken-down protein enters the small intestine from the stomach, stimulating the pancreas to release liquids and enzymes for further breakdown. So it's rather a team effort. Everything in the body has a very specific job and a very specific set of instructions. When you take something out or when something stops working a new management plan must be integrated and taught and that takes time, effort and practice!

Think of your bile as being a bit like washing-up liquid! You have to use it to get the grease off the pan. This is how bile works.

Did you know?

The state of the gallbladder depends greatly on the individual's psychological status.[1] In particular, when a person is upset upon receiving bad news or seeing an accident, the body's first reaction is often an intense contraction of the gallbladder (less often, this may be felt in the stomach). With repetition, this phenomenon can lead to inflammation. This correlation between the psyche and gallbladder applies primarily to superficial psychological tensions; when the problem is deeper and stronger, the entire liver reacts.

ENERGIES OF THE GALLBLADDER

The meridian of the gallbladder

The gallbladder meridian starts at the lateral border of the eye, then travels to the parietal and temporal region of the head, descending along the side of the chest, loin and thigh to the foot and ending near the fourth toe. The gallbladder meridian can affect the gallbladder, the brain, sight and all organs and parts of the body on that side. If the gallbladder meridian is out of balance you can experience gallstones, headaches, migraines, vision problems, dizziness, a stuffy nose, common cold, appendicitis, paralysis and hepatitis.

> ## Properties of the gallbladder meridian
>
> Force: Yang (male)
> Chakra: Solar plexus – personal power, self-will
> Organ body clock: 11pm–1am
> Season: Spring
> Colours: Green
> Fragrances: Sage, carnation and sour aromas
> Metaphysical lesson: Being able to express your willpower,
> feelings of anger and effectively make decisions

The emotions of the gallbladder

The liver and the gallbladder have a relationship that is closer than any other organs in the body. The gallbladder is, surprisingly, a Yang (male) organ, while its best friend the liver is a Yin (female) organ. The gallbladder has a more dominant personality than the liver, so it governs decision-making and planning. An out-of-balance gallbladder comes from not being able to truly express your emotions, or when a person feels invaded by someone close to them in their life, or because they are questioning their place in life and wondering what their purpose is. If the feelings are an unidentifiable frustration, envy and jealousy of others can set in, and if this is the case you can find that people approach this in three different ways: ignore the problem and pretend the solution has been found; cause chaos and create friction by highlighting and elevating the issue (which is a very Yang mentality); or follow a Yin approach by giving in to the feeling and issue and being open about the problem, accepting advice and finding a solution to it. The gallbladder is special in that it is the only organ that does not come into contact with food or drink, unlike the rest of the digestive organs.

THE FOUR BODIES OF THE GALLBLADDER

The spiritual body

The gallbladder is responsible for a person's passion and flow in life and for initiating inspiration for motivation and creativity. When the flow of life feels blocked, stilted or stifled, the gallbladder and its flow of bile can be unbalanced. If you know that there are outstanding issues in your life that need resolving, this imbalance should encourage you to make some changes and tune in to your body and what you need in your life.

Action: Get your creative juices flowing by getting outside and exercising. Neuroscientist Wendy Suzuki, author of *Healthy Brain, Happy Life*[2], states that exercise makes us more creative. BDNF, otherwise known as brain-derived neurotrophic factor, is responsible for brain growth and is stimulated and secreted by the hippocampus of the brain when you are exercising, such as on a long run, a long walk or a long swim. So some time alone outside pumping the cardiovascular system will get rid of those cobwebs and negative thinking and inspire creativity and flow!

The emotional body

You cannot really separate the gallbladder and the liver when it comes to emotions because they feed off each other. Both organs hold similar emotions, with frustration being more specific to the gallbladder. Depression can affect the balance and stability of the gallbladder, because the gallbladder stores bile rather than releasing it and creating flow. When these emotions are strong they can stimulate the sympathetic side of the nervous system and can throw off the balance of the body, making it harder for you to find equilibrium and a sense of calm.

Action: If you recognise that you are overreacting to a situation or you are feeling overwhelmed, step back, take a deep breath, reassess the situation and see if you can find a better solution. Make a note of how you react so you can spot the trigger next time and potentially change your response to a situation.

The nutritional body

Spring is the season of rebirth, renaissance, new beginnings and new life. The colour associated with spring is green and this is the colour we see predominantly in nature, representing new life and growth. This is a time when we can let go of all the negative energy we may have been storing up over the darker winter months. Spring is when all our green vegetables are ready to eat in order to feed our bodies for optimal health. (See seasonal chart on pages 317–21.)

Action: Foods that support the gallbladder are broccoli, rocket, beetroot, basil, garlic, dandelion root, celery, chives and more, because all of these contain sulphur, which stimulates liver detoxification.

The physical body

The meridian of the gallbladder runs bilaterally along the body from the corner of the eye and down the side of the body, ending at the fourth toe, so exercises that stimulate the sides of the body will help the flow of Qi by removing any blockages in the gallbladder organ and meridians. Gallbladders are routinely taken out these days in Western medicine, but in traditional Chinese medicine this would be considered an absolute last resort; they would first look at diet, acupuncture lines, herbs and emotional and nutritional cleanses before removing the most extraordinary organ of the body. In Chinese medicine the health of your emotions is just as important as the food you eat, the amount of sleep you have and the exercise you take.

Action: Tai-chi and qi gong are great internal martial arts for the body, mind and spirit. All movement will prevent the Qi stagnating in the body and in turn will prevent inflammation and disease. Try this exercise:

Stand with your feet wide apart and your hands high in the air. Bend down and touch your right hand on your left foot and come back to standing with your arms in the air and repeat on the other side.

Make sure to twist your body as you touch your toe, creating a rotation around the digestive tract; here you will contract your oblique muscles (the ones at the sides of your body).

Repeat 30 times.

This is a good exercise when you've been sitting down for long periods of time. Try to do it every 45 minutes when you are at work and see how much brighter and creative you feel.

HOW TO LOOK AFTER YOUR GALLBLADDER

Your gallbladder will look after you if you keep compartments of your life organised and clean. Throw out the foods in your cupboards that haven't seen the light of day for a few years and that have really passed their sell-by date. Take any clothes that you have not worn for a year to people who will be able to use them – sometimes these people are closer to home than a charity shop. Give your house a spring-clean, boil your sheets, clean your curtains and steam your carpets.

Nutritional plan for a healthy gallbladder

When the gallbladder is out of balance it struggles to process fatty foods, so avoid any greasy, rich or spicy foods as these will all create discomfort in this organ.

Meals and snacks	Nutrition	Benefits
On waking in the morning	Water and lemon	Detoxifying
First meal of the day	Kombu seaweed and chicken bone broth (see page 81) with 2 garlic cloves and 1 finely chopped red onion	Hydrating and a great way to get your collagen from the chicken broth in an easy-to-digest way. Garlic and onion are antibacterial and anti-inflammatory
Snack, if desired	**Green smoothie:** 1 bunch of parsley 1 apple 3 medium courgettes 225g (8oz) green beans 5 celery sticks	Steam vegetables before blending for better absorption and digestion
Second meal of the day	Dandelion and rocket salad with broccoli and poached cod	Dandelion is a detoxification herb
Snack	Grapefruit segments with stewed apples, walnuts and cinnamon	A sweet/bitter treat to keep you happy
Third meal of the day	Buckwheat pasta with broccoli, pesto and crumbled nuts and seeds	A feel-good meal with the superfood broccoli for its all-round antioxidant effects
Bedtime snack / activity	Dandelion tea leaves	Diuretic

SIGNS THAT YOUR GALLBLADDER IS UNDER STRESS OR UNHAPPY

The signs to look out for to determine if your gallbladder is healthy or not are similar to those you might identify in liver issues – with the exception of the pain-referral patterns. Of course, you may not experience all of these symptoms at one time.

Pain on the right-hand side of the body: You may feel a pain in the right shoulder or neck, or anywhere on the right-hand side of the body. This is because the phrenic nerve, originating from the cervical plexus of vertebrae C3, 4 and 5, feeds the diaphragm. The shoulder is innervated by C5 and when the diaphragm, liver or gallbladder become inflamed it can irritate the supplying dermatome (an area of the skin supplied by nerves from a single spinal root), which creates muscular aches and eventually chronic diffuse pain at the shoulder and neck. A common solution that most people decide upon is to visit a physiotherapist or massage therapist, because this problem presents as muscular or mechanical, but in that situation the etiology will be missed. On speaking with liver surgeon Rafael Ortíz-Rodríguez, of the Nuestra Señora de Candelaria Santa Cruz, in Tenerife (formerly of the Royal Free Hospital in London), he said of the phrenic nerve: 'The phrenic nerve can get irritated with diaphragm irritation. The liver lies close to the diaphragm and the gallbladder lies close to the liver. An inflamed gallbladder could irritate the diaphragm and in turn irritate the phrenic nerve.'

Nausea or fatigue: You may experience some nausea or a sensation that you feel full, which can be symptomatic of the body not being able to efficiently break down fats. Equally, if you are suffering from constipation you may also feel nausea. If these symptoms occur after eating, in particular, it is more likely to be a mechanical biliary problem.

Dyspepsia: Otherwise known as indigestion, this can be experienced after eating fatty foods that the gallbladder does not like; this manifests as a pain in the chest area or stomach. Indigestion can also be a sign of an underlying problem, such as gastro-oesophageal reflux or low hydrochloric acid levels.

Headaches: These tend to start on the left side and slowly spread to the right. They can also turn into migraines.

Stools: Greenish and pale stools are not uncommon but they are also not normal. You will produce green stools either because you have eaten food with green food colourings or because the bile has not had time to break down your food and the transit time has been too quick. You may notice this colouration when you have diarrhoea.

Dandelion for the gallbladder

Dandelion extract: Dandelion – both the root and leaf – is a classic bitter detoxification tonic herb, as it stimulates digestion and stimulates the liver to produce more bile. This action cleanses the liver and gallbladder.

Fun fact from Bill Bryson: 'The dandelion was popularly known as the "pissabed" because of its supposed diuretic properties and other names in everyday use included "mare's fats", "naked ladies", "twitch bollock", "hound piss", "open arse" and "bum towel".'[3]

Top ingredients for your gallbladder

Celery seed: This protects against as well as reverses the effects of acetaminophen on the liver, which is analgesic. As a diuretic it also helps flush out toxins. Dip a quail's egg into celery seed, it's yummy!

Chicory (*Cichorium intybus*): This cholagogic food helps stimulate bile flow. It is a bitter and versatile leaf that can be eaten raw – you can add to salads, and it has a beautiful pink colouring. The root can be ground and used as chicory root coffee, although it doesn't really compare to the bean!

Mustard greens: Perfect for a spring lunch: sauté in olive oil with crushed garlic and finely chopped onions and drizzle with a touch of basil-infused oil.

Cucumber, basil and lemon water: This is hydrating, immunity-boosting and easy to prepare. Simply cold-press the juice of half a cucumber with the juice of half a lemon, add four large basil leaves and drink.

FAT: A FEARED PLEASURE

Fat is vogue; it is a subject that is discussed and debated endlessly, but if you're eating the right type and the right amount of it, it should not make you fat. Fat is the macronutrient that stops you continuously thinking about food, satisfies your hunger hormones and allows you to get on with your day. Being on a diet of sorts has become the norm for many people these days, and in our quest for the body beautiful we cut out fat, the effect of which is that we then have to endure emotional outbursts, erratic behaviour and indecision.

The reason why fat can make you fat is simply down to the fact that it contains 9 calories per gram, whereas carbohydrates and protein contain 4 calories per gram. However, as we have learnt from Gary Taubes (on pages 8–9), calories in versus calories out was one of the most damaging statements for health in history.

Our relationship with weight, with fat and with food affects everything in our lives. The fat we eat makes us happy, it makes food taste good, and when you opt for the low-fat option you sacrifice not only taste but also pleasure. There is only so much pleasure a low-fat chocolate eclair can give you, because rather than satisfying you with fat it drugs you with sugar. And that's the difference: sugar is like a friend who is there one minute and gone the next. Fat commits to the relationship.

Take away the fat and you have to increase the sugar, which is counterproductive.

I do not see a world getting thinner because they have given up fat – far from it. We only have three macronutrients (the other two being protein and carbohydrates) and they are all equally important for the health of the body, so cutting out one seems like a rather bad idea to me, and one that creates more problems than it solves.

We have swapped butter for margarine, lard for vegetable oil, we cut the white bits off the meat wherever we can, we go for fat-free products if possible and we punish ourselves with low-fat dressings, low-fat cakes, zero-fat milk and zero-fat yoghurt – all in search of the body beautiful and the taste-free life. If we do overindulge we pull out all the stops to redress the calorific intake by stopping eating for a day or grazing on lattes and cappuccinos until we make it to the darkest hour. Then, of course, we simply climb into the fridge at midnight and here, out of sight and out of mind, we shamefully stuff our faces, because tomorrow is another day when we can start again and, more importantly, if no one saw me it didn't happen. When did eating lose its pleasurable qualities?

The war on saturated fat is one of the biggest mistakes in the history of nutrition.

People with type 2 diabetes have an inability to utilise glucose/sugar through loss of insulin sensitivity or inability of the cells to utilise carbohydrates. Sugars come from carbohydrates, so you might think that advising someone with diabetes to follow a high-carbohydrate, low-fat diet would be a preposterous idea, but in fact until the 1980s that was the official advice.

In the 1950s, respected American nutritionist Ancel Benjamin Keys, a biologist and pathologist, supposedly showed that animal fat was the main cause of heart disease because it clogged up the arteries.[4] Everyone was advised to cut their fat intake, including diabetics, on the grounds that they were at an increased risk of heart disease. Keys' theory rested on three main points: that low-fat diets kept the arteries clearer and so protected the heart, made it easier to lose weight – because gram for gram fat had twice as many calories as carbohydrates – and reduced the level of lipids (fats) in the blood.

Keys supported his theory with data he had gathered on coronary heart disease and fat consumption from seven countries.[5] The research he published, though, only concluded what he had found in seven countries where fat and cholesterol were high, as was the risk of dying from heart disease. Later research showed that picking a different seven countries showed no connection.

But that made no difference to the official policy, nor did research by British nutrition expert Professor John Yudkin, who put the blame for heart disease on sugar. The success of Dr Atkins' low-carb, high-fat weight-loss diet in the 1980s and 1990s was also ignored. But in recent years doctors and scientists have begun to realise that fat has been wrongly demonised, including an international expert on carbohydrates, Professor Richard Feinman of New York University, whose team found that fat, in fact, makes people feel fuller than carbs and so they eat less.[6] Today the advice from the NHS website for people with diabetes is to 'choose foods that are low in fat – replace butter, ghee and coconut oil with low-fat spreads and vegetable oil, choose skimmed and semi-skimmed milk, and low-fat yoghurts'.[7] And so the contradiction continues to live on.

Fat: victims of the war on fat

Fats technically called lipids have historically had a lot of bad press, being cited as the reason why we are fat, have high cholesterol and blood pressure, diabetes, insulin resistance, etc. So let's break down fat groupings and concentrate on the good ones.

Fat comes in a few shapes and sizes; however, the main ones are saturated fats, polyunsaturated fats and monounsaturated fats.

Saturated fats: mainly found in animal products and coconut.

Polyunsaturated fats: mainly found in plant and animal foods as well as nuts and seeds.

Monounsaturated fats: mainly found in avocados, olive oil and nuts.

Trans fats (artificial): mainly found in processed foods. These are created by an industrial process which makes them very difficult for your body to break down.

The best fats for a healthy body

Good fats	Type of fat	What it does
Coconut oil	Saturated fat Medium-chain fatty acid	Coconut oil is a stable oil which is solid at room temperature and has a melting point of 25°C (77°F). It's made up of 50 per cent lauric acid and this has antimicrobial properties. It is anti-inflammatory and the fatty acids help the brain and memory functions
Butter; grass-fed and organic	Saturated fat Low smoke point, so best not to cook directly with this	Real butter, not margarine or butter spread – real butter from an organically reared cow. Perfect mix of omega 3 and 6; arachidonic acid helps with brain function, skin health and prostaglandin balance. Also a source of selenium, a strong antioxidant
Olive oil/ Extra virgin olive oil in a glass bottle	Monounsaturated	Olive oil is rich in monounsaturated fat, which research suggests helps prevent or slow down the cognitive decline associated with diseases like Alzheimer's[8]

Avocado	Monounsaturated	Avocados are particularly rich in potassium, even higher than the often-touted bananas, and a good food to eat for normal blood pressure and a lower risk of kidney failure and heart disease
Ghee; clarified butter (Indian version of butter)	Saturated fat Perfect for high temperatures	Ghee stimulates the secretion of gastric acid, thus aiding the digestive process. It is also lactose- and casein-free. High in k2, which will help strengthen your bones

Setting the record straight: a few things you need to know about cholesterol

Cholesterol for years has been at the forefront of many a health debate. Cholesterol is made in the liver and is an essential ingredient for hormones, delivered via the bloodstream.

- Cholesterol is made predominantly in the liver, with a small amount coming from the lining of the intestines.
- Avoiding foods high in saturated fats and rich in cholesterol will not decrease the prevalence of heart disease, as they contain nutrients essential for heart health. However, avoiding trans fats is beneficial.
- Cholesterol is one of the most important molecules in your body; it is indispensable for the building of cells and for producing stress and sex hormones, as well as providing vitamin D.

Total cholesterol tells you virtually nothing about your heart-disease risk. However, NMR LipoProfile, HDL/cholesterol ratio and triglyceride/HDL ratio offer more accurate risk assessments. Your doctor or health-care practitioner will be able to explain what each of these mean.

PATHOLOGIES OF THE GALLBLADDER

Gallstones (Cholelithiasis)

Gallstones are the bane of the gallbladder and the major cause of the removal of this organ (called a cholecystectomy). One or more calculi (gallstones) will be present in the gallbladder, usually made of cholesterol or crystallised bile of the common bile duct. Gallstones come in two forms: the most common, cholesterol stones, account for 80 per cent of gallstone cases and are usually yellow-green in colour. Then there are pigment stones, which are smaller, darker and made up of bilirubin, which comes from bile.

Gallstones are not to be taken lightly, because complications can arise if they are not treated correctly, resulting in cholecystitis, jaundice, acute cholangitis, acute pancreatitis or even gallbladder cancer.

In developed countries at least 10–20 per cent of adults and over 20 per cent of people over 65 years old have gallstones. Common side-effects are usually pain, nausea or inflammation in the body. Gallstones become particularly troublesome when they travel down the common bile duct all the way to the junction with the pancreatic duct and beyond. The pain can be excruciating, much like the intensity of urinating when you have cystitis. The gallstones can become stuck and form a blockage, which, as you can imagine, intensifies the pain, but not only that, it can also lead to infection, lesions and even breakage of the duct (the last one is very rare). The condition is called choledocholithiasis and always requires medical treatment, or at the very least some advice. Sufferers complain of sporadic and unpredictable episodes that are localised to the epigastrium or right upper quadrant, sometimes radiating to the right scapular tip.

The number of gallbladder surgeries performed in the last five years has certainly increased, as the technique has become easier. Studies estimate that removals have risen from 22 to 57 per cent during the first year since the introduction of the new procedure, which involves using a laparoscope as a camera which is inserted via long instruments through small holes in the tummy. According to the National Institute for Health and Care Excellence (NICE), 66,000 cholecystectomies are performed every year in the UK with gallbladder surgery now about as common as a hysterectomy, which is second only to Caesarean sections. But is a cholecystectomy a solution? The answer to that is, yes, it is if there is a blockage in the pancreatic duct, which could potentially lead to pancreatitis and is life-threatening. However, if this is not the case then there are other solutions like diet, supplementation, lifestyle – all factors that need to be at the heart of a wellness programme as they are then foundations of health and they should at the very least be reviewed before succumbing to the surgeon's knife. So it is a positive thought to know that surgery is not always the only option and it just requires some research and advice and a good look at you, your body, lifestyle and diet so you can change what is not working and improve on what is.

All these cholecystectomies beg a couple of questions: Why is this modern-day illness on the rise and why is this rise highest among youngsters? Dr Thomas H. Lewis, a board-certified surgeon and a Fellow in the American College of Surgeons, suggests that perhaps modern-day fad diets are to blame, as people lose too much weight too quickly.[9] Women are more at risk and genetics can also play a role, he says. Perhaps the real reason why we have more of a chole cystectomy prevalence these days, especially among the young, is down to oestrogen and endocrine disruptors. Oestrogen is a female steroid hormone responsible for reproduction. Oestrogen dominance is more common now than ever before, with conditions such as endometriosis, uterine fibroids, PCOS, PMS and breast cancers on the rise. Oestrogen excess can increase cholesterol and bile production, which can be the cause of gallstones. A healthy diet keeps our oestrogen levels low and gallstones away but endocrine disrupters like beauty and household products with chemicals and parabens in them (see page 32) and chemicals added to our food all mimic oestrogen. The oestrogen is then stored in the adipose tissues making us fatter and the cells resistant to change.

The good news is that all this can be avoided with natural foods, filtered water, regular exercise, paraben-free beauty products and household cleaning products.

When a gallbladder is removed you take away the physical body but the energetic function still remains.

Case study

The female touch

Emily was referred to me by a male colleague who thought she needed the 'female touch'. He described her as anxious and frantic and, indeed, she was to become the most anxious client I have dealt with.

Complaining of pain in her ribs and uncomfortable wind problems, she was convinced that bile was leaking into her stomach. She needed constant reassurance and support – both practical and emotional. I sent Emily to a visceral manipulator to check the direction of the pyloric sphincter (which lies between the stomach and the small intestines), as a frozen or displaced sphincter can disrupt the flow of substances, which was the case with Emily. Her oesophagus, liver and gallbladder were also flagged as being in a sympathetic state and she had a hiatus hernia.

In addition, she had an inverted breathing pattern, which was contributing to her overall stress levels.

On consultation, the gallbladder surgeon recommended a gallbladder removal because it was only functioning at 35 per cent. However, by this time there were positive changes in Emily and she was eating a wider variety of foods – previously she had been restricted to just chicken and carrots, but now she was able to introduce more greens and fish. She told me her joints would ache when she didn't eat, so to assist digestion we added Lypo Gold enzymes into her diet to help fat breakdown, and B12 for absorption.

One of her issues was bile reflux. This occurs when bile escapes into the oesophagus when there is a weakening or abnormal relaxing of the muscular valve which allows food to pass into the stomach. This can be caused by a peptic ulcer blocking the pyloric valve, so it doesn't open enough to allow the stomach to empty as quickly as it should. As a result, stagnant food in the stomach leads to increased gastric pressure and makes it more likely for bile and stomach acid to back up into the oesophagus.

People who have had their gallbladders removed have significantly more bile reflux than people who haven't had this surgery, so obviously Emily wasn't keen on the surgical option. I suggested bringing in Gall Plus by Nutri Advanced; black radish complex, a specialised complex containing bile salts; glandulars (a supplement for damaged organs and tissues); and other nutrients and herbs, all of which can help support the health of the liver and gallbladder and assist in the emulsification and absorption of dietary fats. By December 2015, Emily was a lot calmer and less anxious, eating more foods and feeling happier in herself.

Healing options after a cholecystectomy

If you have had a cholecystectomy or decide to have one, you must make sure you are supporting your digestive capability's fat breakdown with good nutrition and supplementation. If you do this, you will be able to support this removal; if you don't, you may well find that you begin to have some painful episodes, digestive cramps and bowel issues. There are many steps you can take to make sure you look after your health as best you can (see box below).

Solution	Why
Take digestive enzymes	These are the secret ingredients to perfect digestion; these are made in a few organs – namely the stomach, the pancreas and small intestine and can be depleted, making digestion harder.
Bitter foods	Bitter foods such as rocket, dandelion greens, dill, Jerusalem artichoke and kale stimulate digestive enzymes, so try to get these into your breakfast, lunch and dinner at least once a day.
Juice vegetables	Juicing allows you to get the vital minerals and vitamins into your body without too much digestion. Perfect when you need the nutrients but lack the energy to break them down, i.e. after surgery.
Supplements	**Milk thistle tincture** is a great tonic for the liver, improving and regenerating liver cells and the solubility of bile. Take 15–20 drops twice a day. **Sunflower lecithin** – take 1–2 capsules with food. This breaks down fats and makes them easier to digest, and helps cholesterol to move through the bloodstream. **Vitamin C** is required for the conversion of cholesterol into bile salts. The UK RDA is 60mg; you can also get this by eating oranges, red peppers, kiwis, and brightly coloured fruit and veg in general. **Taurine, glutamine and glycine** reduce the inflammation of the liver and gallbladder (do not take glutamine if you have cancer). **Bile salts** – 1–3 capsules with fatty meals to help digest fats.

Other ways to help yourself through a cholecystectomy

Socialise with friends: See friends and keep busy; make sure you have a social event with good friends each week to look forward to.

Self-love: Put yourself as your top priority. You are the most important person in your life. Take time for you to rest and repair; it's an essential requirement to being awesome!

Rest: Take some time out to rest. Book the week off work at least. Catch up on your favourite box set, read that book you got for Christmas, but take it easy.

Exercise: The best exercise you can do over this time is walking outside. It's a bonus if you can walk in the country, otherwise going to the local park or around the block has wonderful physical as well as mental benefits.

High cholesterol (Hypercholesterolaemia)

Cholesterol gets a bad reputation when you have too many fatty deposits in your blood vessels (atheroma/atherosclerosis), which can indeed increase your chance of heart disease. But it is in fact vital for cell formation, vitamin D and certain hormones. Cholesterol is a waxy, fat-like substance that can come from your diet, but the majority is produced by your liver and excreted by the bile from your gallbladder. The key to having the right amount for you is making sure that you get the right fats from your food and look after your nutrition.

Cholesterol is amphiphatic and it doesn't easily dissolve in water so it can't travel through the body by itself. Lipoproteins help transport the cholesterol through the bloodstream. There are two major forms of these:

LDL, low-density lipoprotein, mainly carries cholesterol from the liver to the cells of the body. Its street name is Bad Cholesterol: it's basically the stuff you don't want and the first figure you look at when you get your blood tests back. LDL has a hard job because it has to carry the cholesterol around, and if it gets too full with cholesterol some may fall out when travelling down the arteries, causing a blockage.

HDL, the high-density lipoprotein, on the other hand, has a good reputation and, much like the head girl at school, can't do anything wrong. She dutifully collects the cholesterol from the cells and transports it to the liver where it is either used, excreted through the bile or converted into bile salts.

> **What you're looking for when you get your cholesterol checked is the optimal ranges of cholesterol:**
>
> - Total cholesterol less than 5 mmol/litre.
> - LDL cholesterol less than 3 mmol/litre.
> - Triglycerides less than 1.7 mmol/litre.
> - HDL cholesterol over 1mmol/litre.

Statins are often prescribed if your cholesterol levels are out of range. These work by preventing the liver making cholesterol, but a side-effect is that they also cause muscle pain.

Reasons why you may have high cholesterol

High cholesterol typically doesn't come with any symptoms but can be the cause of other issues. High cholesterol has caused plaque to build up in the arteries, so the arteries are thus narrower so that less blood can flow through them, which changes your arterial lining, leading to more serious situations such as heart attacks, strokes and coronary heart disease.

A family history: If you have a family history of high cholesterol you are more likely to have high cholesterol yourself, so you may need to get your cholesterol levels checked regularly. Talk to your doctor about your personal condition.

Genetic link: There is a genetic condition called familial hypercholesterolaemia which is passed through genes. People with this condition have cholesterol levels of 300mg/dl or higher. They may also develop xanthoma, which is the appearance of a yellow patch under the skin.

Smoking: Smoking reduces lung capacity; by stopping you reduce your chances of developing cancer by over 30 per cent. Smoking raises your chances of coronary heart disease, especially if you already have cholesterol issues.

Excess alcohol consumption: Alcohol puts strain on the heart by altering the rhythm of the heartbeat (arrhythmia), which can lead to heart muscle disease (cardiomyopathy). It increases and maintains high blood pressure, causes obesity and increases triglycerides and cholesterol.

What high cholesterol might look or feel like to you
Being overweight: If you carry your weight around your waist you could be increasing your chances of high triglyceride levels and therefore high cholesterol and atherosclerosis. Women should aim for a waist circumference of less than 80cm (31½ inches) and men should be less than 94cm (37 inches). If you are overweight this will undoubtedly put more stress on the body and its organs, so getting your body back into balance will make it more efficient.

Broken capillaries on the face: Sometimes referred to as spider veins, this can occur when blood pressure is high, which can be symptomatic of high cholesterol and another reason to get this checked out with the doctor.

Shortness of breath: If the arteries have narrowed in response to high cholesterol you might find yourself out of breath, so it's worth getting a check-up with the doctor.

WHY BREATHING AND POSTURE ARE KINGS

I'd like to discuss two more things before we leave the gallbladder behind and move on to the kidneys. To ensure your gallbladder and all your organs are working properly, you need to breathe properly and have good posture. Sounds simple, right? But you'd be surprised how many of us, particularly with regard to breathing, aren't utilising the full force of our lungs.

Breathing is the hierarchy to all bodily systems and functions. It can create health and it can deplete it and create a toxic environment.

Breathing can change the pH in the body, just as the pH can affect your breathing. The normal pH in the body is 7.35–7.45. Respiratory alkalosis is due to the increased rate of breathing, which decreases the amount of carbon dioxide and hydrogen in the body. When these two compounds are eliminated from the body too quickly it increases the pH level. The heart and kidneys are greatly affected, thus abnormalities in emotional status and endocrine systems follow.

Diet and posture can also shift the balance. Making poor food choices can increase breathing due to the inflammatory responses in the mucosal lining which constricts the airways. A very common theme is to subconsciously move the head forwards to improve the capacity to breathe. This is detrimental to the body because the body's survival mechanism is to maintain vision and eye level on the horizon. Cranial extension (backward tilt of the skull) is the outcome that can create ischaemia and limit healthy oxygenated blood to the brain due to the path of the vertebral arteries. The vertebral arteries extend from the subclavian artery, run up the lateral aspects of the cervical spine from C6, wrap around the posterior arch of the atlas (C1) and into the brain stem.

Coupled with forward head posture comes a depression or downward tilt of the ribcage. This downward tilt of the ribcage and forward bending of the thoracic spine limits full excursion of the diaphragm. When the lungs expand during inhalation the diaphragm is driven downward. Upon exhalation the diaphragm is driven upwards. When posture is compromised oxygen uptake is limited and the sympathetic nervous system is activated. Many bodily functions and chemical pathways are changed.

Also with forward head posture and changes in the spinal angles come emotional problems, such as anxiety, panic attacks and stress, due to the link to limited movement of the diaphragm.

The diaphragm is very important in keeping a strong rigid foundation for the shoulder to work from during overhead activities. Due to the pendulous nature of the arms when the ribcage, thoracic spine, cervical spine and cranium migrate forwards, the shoulder sits in a forward position that changes the tension relationships between the muscles around the shoulder during static and dynamic movement. Pain and joint destruction are resultant; the chest muscles will start to shorten and may create trigger points, pain patterns, and simulate heart-attack symptoms such as pain running down the arm.

Posture is the passive rest position of the musculoskeletal system. It is where movement starts and finishes. Optimal posture is keeping the ear, shoulder, hip, knee and ankle in line.

Posture and digestive discomfort

Poor posture inhibits the mobility of the internal organs in three dimensions. Organs like bones have ligamentous joints and when the joints are underused, fascial (connective tissue) restrictions (tightness) and inflammation occur. The movement of organs is predominantly affected by breathing and posture; if posture is poor, the health of the organs will be poor, too. Think of Superman: he had good posture – tall and upright with a strong chest and his head on his shoulders, which creates room for his organs as good posture creates space for them. Now think of a sluggish posture, with hips forward and head forward. This sway-back posture promotes a forward head posture and a depression in the diaphragm and ribs, where many of your organs are housed. This then poses the question: does your GI discomfort stem from your poor posture?

Movement for your organs

The body is made up of bones, muscles, nerves and a thin connective tissue called fascia, as well as the internal organs (viscera). Your organs are in perpetual motion – for instance when you breathe and when you move.

Visceral mobility is the health prescription that is needed for healthy and functional organs, and it is important because mobility creates good circulation. Poor blood circulation can affect the function of the organ as all organs are fed by blood. If a person does not have good visceral mobility they may have poor posture, which can affect the shape of the thorax and the abdomen, thereby squashing the organs, which results in decreased movement.

Poor mobility can also be a result of the GIT inflammatory process. In between the fascia membranes of each viscera is a serous fluid that enables organs to move freely – the heart beats, the lungs expand, the stomach and the intestines contract and the bladder empties. It is the space in between the fluid and the viscera where the inflammatory process starts and this is what creates the adhesions on the viscera, which is how you get infections.

A bacterial or parasitic infection, for example, can create a stickiness between the fascial envelopes. The fascia functions as a joint and the organ articulates around that fascial restriction, so when you have an adhesion from one organ to the next it creates another axis on which that organ rotates, so the adhesions become a false articulation for that organ. For example, the liver rotates in three dimensions around the left and right triangular ligaments if you have an adhesion to the diaphragm, and rather than the liver articulating around those two points you now have a third point, which messes up the articulation and mobility of the organ. So you can begin to see that the effects of fascial adhesion are problematic and it can be deep-rooted in gastro health, but affect all the organs of the body.

Dr Jean-Pierre Barral found the following correlations through his work in visceral manipulation[10]:

Issue or condition	Reason for the pain
Frozen shoulder	Nerve irritation stemming from the visceral pleura
Right shoulder pain	Restriction in your liver
Chronically cold feet	Issues in the small intestines
Heartburn/gastric reflux	Stomach sitting too high

TOP 10 TIPS FOR A HEALTHY GALLBLADDER

1. **Steam your greens:** Steaming rather than boiling is the best way to eat your greens hot, as this method of cooking maximises vitamin and nutrient uptake.

2. **Bitters:** These are a combination of various bitter-tasting herbs which serve as a tonic for overall vitality while specifically enhancing digestive health. Bitters begin to do their work the moment they touch your tongue. Their bitter nature stimulates the stomach, the liver, the gallbladder and the pancreas to begin secreting vital digestive components used to assimilate nutrients in the body, such as bile, gastric juices and insulin. The liver's ability to eliminate toxins is also enhanced.

3. **Do yoga:** Yoga has been perfectly designed for the health and movement of your organs; when we breathe we give our organs a workout

and this is what is taught in yoga. Start with some gentle hatha yoga if you are a beginner.

4. **Eat good clean fats:** Despite popular opinion, a low-fat diet is not the best option if you are suffering with gallstones as it puts more stress on the liver, which is having to work hard to break down carbohydrates.

5. **Avoid trans fats:** It is critical to avoid all fried foods, especially if they are bought from a shop or restaurant because they can reheat the oils for cooking, making them even more unstable and carcinogenic. Make sure you read your labels – avoid all types of fats that are hydrogenated, partially hydrogenated or are trans fats. Fats that are not natural are hard, if not impossible, for your body to break down, so they will create toxicity and problems for your digestive system but also put pressure on your gallbladder and liver.

6. **Decrease alcohol consumption:** Alcohol is not a good friend of the gallbladder or the liver. You have to be aware of the consequences: if you put too many toxins in the body, with no repair management, the gallbladder will create gallstones and can potentially get blocked and cause a lot of pain.

7. **Chew your food:** Chewing your food is the first part of digestion, and the first thing I tell my clients is that if you are not chewing, the enzymes from the salivary amylase are not produced efficiently and food breakdown is impaired, potentially leading to digestive symptoms of bloating and gas.

8. **Give up processed food for good:** There is no benefit to eating food that is not from this earth. If Mother Nature has not created it, your body does not have the enzymes to break it down. It is that simple. Only the big guy in *James Bond* ('Jaws', aka Richard Kiel) was able to do this efficiently! Stick to what nature intended; if it grew from the ground, fell off a bush or a tree, or has a pair of eyes, it's yours to eat. If you can't figure out how it got to being on your plate, you should probably dispose of it, as your body won't be able to!

9. **Add garlic and onions:** Super-duper cleansers for the gallbladder.

When these are both eaten raw they have fantastic healing properties. Both are antibacterial and antiparasitic.

10. **Squeeze your lemons:** This is the best tonic for the gallbladder. Lemon juice and other juices high in citric acid and vitamin C have been used by themselves or combined with olive oil and Epsom salts to reduce calcifications in the gallbladder and kidneys for many generations. Once in the blood, citric acid and vitamin C can dissolve certain types of calcifications in the body.

Footnotes

(1) Barral, J.-P., *Visceral Manipulation* (California, 2008).

(2) Suzuki, W., *Healthy Brain, Happy Life* (New York, 2015).

(3) Bryson, B., *A Short History of Nearly Everything* (London, 2003).

(4) Keys, A., 'The seven countries study', www.sevencountriesstudy.com (accessed on 25/01/2016).

(5) Keys, A., 'Coronary heart disease in seven countries. Summary', *Circulation* (Waltham, 1970).

(6) Feinman, R., 'Dietary carbohydrate restriction as the first approach in diabetes management: critical review and evidence base', *Nutrition* (New York, 2015).

(7) NHS Choices, Type 2 Diabetes, www.nhs.uk/conditions/type-2-diabetes/treatment/ (accessed on 21/01/2018).

(8) Gonzalez, G., Marcos, A., Pietzik, K., 'Nutrition and cognitive impairment in the elderly', *British Journal of Nutrition* (Cambridge, 2007).

(9) Lewis, T., 'Gallbladder Disease – A Modern Illness on the Rise', www.bmhvt.org/gallbladder-disease-modern-illness-rise/ (accessed on 21/01/2016).

(10) Barral, J.-P., *Understanding the Messages of Your Body: How to Interpret Physical and Emotional Signals to Achieve Optimal Health* (California, 2008).

4. THE KIDNEYS

Fear

They are called the gifts of life; everyone can donate a kidney and continue to live a perfectly healthy life while saving that of another. The average wait for a kidney transplant in the UK is 15 years, making kidneys the most sought-after organs in the human body. It is the ultimate gift.

And why are they so precious? Kidneys are the cleaners of the body, working around the clock, pumping and cleaning. It would be easy to take the kidneys for granted, but you shouldn't because if they do fail they won't give you any warning signs. Dialysis offers a life extension, but not a full life, so it's better to treat your kidneys kindly and take simple preventative measures to avoid kidney failure.

Your kidneys are a pair of dark-red, bean-shaped, fist-sized organs that sit just below your ribcage and under your adrenal glands, on either side of the posterior wall of the abdominal cavity. The left kidney is located slightly higher than the right kidney because the right side of the liver is much larger than the left. The kidneys are retroperitoneal, meaning they sit between the dorsal wall and the peritoneum, the membrane that surrounds the abdominal cavity. A layer of adipose (fat) tissues holds the kidneys in place and protects them against physical damage.

You could almost compare the kidneys to the latest washer and drier, except the kidneys would iron, too! They are a feature-packed, quality cleaning service with high-speed filtration, reabsorption and secretion. The kidneys keep stock of some high-quality sought-after vitamins and hormones and are confined, compliant, compact, self-contained and favourably low maintenance.

If you compare the amount of work that the kidneys undertake every hour of every day in comparison to their size, you'd be amazed. They have such a strong work ethic, we could learn a thing or two from the kidneys! On a daily basis, 1,500 litres (2,640 pints) of blood passes through them, efficiently travelling through an intricate terrain, through pumps and channels that make sure two essential processes happen: nutrients are absorbed and waste products are excreted in volumes of up to 2 litres (3½ pints) in the form of urine, your pee.

Kidney facts:

- Kidneys clean your blood and are responsible for removing waste products like carbon dioxide from the body.
- In a single hour, the kidneys receive around 180 litres (317 pints) of blood to filter.
- They are full of blood, which is what makes them look so red.
- Throughout the day, the kidneys filter and produce around 1–2 litres (1¾–3½ pints) of urine, but on average we excrete around 1.5 litres (2½ pints) of urine in a single day.

A BIT MORE ANATOMY

The kidneys are part of the renal system, along with the two ureters, bladder and urethra. The renal system has all sorts of important jobs to perform, such as regulating water volume, ion salts and pH levels, as well as influencing your red blood cell production and blood pressure. Its main job is concerned with filtering toxic leftovers from the blood, such as nitrogenous waste made by metabolising proteins, and driving it out of the body. So it's not just your digestive system that has to deal with the aftermath of the food and liquid that you eat, we should also be paying homage to these fine masters of their art – the blood-red kidneys and the rest of the renal system.

There are two ureters, each 25–30 centimetres (10–12 inches) long, which run on the left- and right-hand sides of the vertebral column, and their job is to carry urine from the kidneys to the bladder. There are valves at the end of the ureters to stop the urine flowing back up towards the kidneys.

At any moment your kidneys hold 20 per cent of the total blood volume of the body.

The bladder is another holding sac similar to the stomach and the gall-bladder – hollow, distensible and muscular – with a similar function to the stomach. The bladder stores urine, while the stomach stores hydrochloric acid. You can locate the bladder at the inferior end of the pelvis – at your belly button, go down 5 centimetres (2 inches) and exert a light pressure and you will feel your bladder; if it is full it may be slightly uncomfortable and sensitive. As urine comes down from the ureters it fills the bladder. The elastic walls of the bladder expand to hold anything from 600–800 millilitres (21–28 fl oz) of urine at a time.

The urethra is a tube that extends from the bladder to the exterior of the body, transporting and expelling urine. The female urethra is around 5 centimetres (2 inches) long and ends behind the clitoris and above the vaginal opening. The urethra in males is 20–25 centimetres (8–10 inches) long and ends at the tip of the penis. The male urethra also carries sperm out of the body through the penis. The flow of urine through the urethra is controlled by the sphincter muscles, both internal and external. When the bladder reaches a level of dis-tention the internal sphincter opens at the same time or hopefully just before you have the sensation to urinate. When you feel the sensation to pee but are not in the appropriate place to do so, the external sphincter, made of skeletal muscle, will close to make sure there are no embarrassing moments.

The kidneys perform their life-sustaining job of filtering and reabsorbing over 200 litres (352 pints) of fluid every day – some of which is excreted as urine. The urine that is to be excreted is stored in the bladder for up to 10 hours, which is why you will either go to the toilet in the middle of the night or first thing in the morning.

Did you know?

Iran is the only country in the world where you can legally sell a kidney for profit. It is estimated 1,400 Iranians sell a kidney every year. The Iranian board of ministers approved it in 1997 and today there are no waiting lists for kidney transplants. Not all kidneys are accepted, however, and some say the initiative exploits the poor and vulnerable.

ENERGIES OF THE KIDNEYS

The meridian of the kidneys

The kidney meridian starts at the sole of the foot and ascends along the outside of the leg, through the thigh, the abdomen and the sternum to the clavicle. An unbalanced kidney meridian can manifest physically in the feet, groin area and/or diaphragm. When the kidney meridian is out of balance, women may have irregular periods, or reproductive issues. It can contribute to constipation, hypertension and the hiccups.

It could be said that the kidneys are the workhorses of the body and that a person who displays traits of hard work and strength, especially for long periods of time, will have strong kidneys and will be full of power and determination, will be good at making decisions and have an intuitive nature. However, sometimes these people can try to do everything for themselves and not ask for help. They may have been let down in the past or experienced a trauma where they now only rely on themselves and this can lead to a weak kidney energy. The kidneys work in conjunction with your adrenal glands and with a weak energy the adrenal glands can be suffering. They may try to rectify this by excessive behaviours such as over-exercise, addictions or increased sexual activity, eating high-sugar foods and avoiding trying to achieve their goal or dream. Weak energies are also associated with fear, anxiety and change in life and so can often spend long periods of time in their own space.

The kidneys love water

In traditional Chinese medicine the kidneys are closely related to fear. It is important to remember that the mind and the spirit have a close connection in the body that cannot be separated. When there is an imbalance in the kidneys, thoughts of fear can set in and cause more disruption. The kidneys are also closely linked with the adrenals and the reproductive system, so any imbalance in the kidneys can also cause these systems to fall out of balance.

Properties of the kidney meridian

Force: Yin (female)

Chakra: Sacral plexus – sexuality and creativity

Organ body clock: 5–7pm

Season: Winter

Colours: Black and yellow

Fragrances: Mint and orange

Metaphysical lesson: Self anger and fear

The emotions of the kidneys

Fear is a normal and adaptive human emotion. We all experience fear, but when the perceived cause of fear is not dealt with or addressed it can lead to an imbalance in our emotional status, because emotions and organs are connected. Generations ago you could argue there was much more reason to be fearful; worrying about where the next meal came from, how the rent would be paid, if there would be an air raid or enough rations, or news of a death on the battlefield. Today our fears are very different, and not always so life-threatening, and yet we drop happy pills and sleeping pills like popcorn at the cinema to cope with our fear-injected lifestyles.

There was no class at school to teach us how to assess risk, chance or emotional intelligence, but there should have been. Being felled by fear is as common as being constipated. Fear manifests itself in everyday stressors; it is relative and today we may have money worries, anxiety over buying a house, finding the right partner, growing old, looking after family or having sick relatives to contend with – then if you add the social media frenzy into the mix, which brings anxiety over being liked, being funny, hanging out with the in-crowd, being seen, posting videos, getting into the magazines, etc., it's no wonder that we are all so stressed out. The health and fitness world also puts fear on a pedestal, which is detrimental to our health and wellbeing.

Fear is one of the most commonly felt emotions.

THE FOUR BODIES OF THE KIDNEYS

The spiritual body

All the substances that enter the bloodstream have to pass through a 'selection' process via the kidneys. When the kidneys are out of balance, so too is our judgement and our ability to make decisions.

As the kidneys are put under pressure through the filtering process, our ability to filter past and present situations and environments becomes harder, and our abilities to reason and be discerning reduces.

The kidneys are filters. They decide what you need and what you don't through a highly efficient system called glomerular filtration. By the end of the cleaning process the kidneys will have filtered all the fluids that belong to the human body, which represent 60–75 per cent of the weight of an adult body.

Action: It is important to detach yourself from past behaviours that do not fit your present time and to try to master your emotions so that your old beliefs do not hold you back in life and you are not governed by fear. In order to do this, start by listing on paper the traits that do not serve you to see if there is a pattern in your behaviour. Are you always going back to learn the same lesson because you have not established what you need to learn?

The emotional body

According to traditional Chinese medicine, the kidneys' positive characteristics are wisdom, rationality, gentleness and understanding, and on the negative side are fear, loneliness, insecurity and shock. The kidneys contain the criticism, disappointment and failures bestowed upon us. They are intimately related to fear, low self-esteem, insecurities and apathy for the present moment, isolation and indifference. The kidneys, particularly the adrenal glands, are especially vulnerable to damage from excessive stress, over-exercise and emotional trauma.

Action: Strengthen the energy of the kidneys with acupuncture and traditional Chinese herbs to help self-esteem and strengthen the ji qing line associated with strong kidneys.

The nutritional body

The job of the kidneys is to keep the body's fluids and electrolytes in a healthy balance. The kidneys love water, so make sure that above all else they get at least 1.5 litres (2½ pints) of water every day. If they are well hydrated you will feel better, sleep better, look better and move better. The typical Western diet is not a friend of the kidneys and is in fact the reason why we see a high prevalence of kidney stones, with a diet high in trans fats and saturated fats, processed meats and refined sugars. In countries where fibre intake is high there is much less prevalence of kidney stones.

Magnesium-rich foods: All dark leafy green vegetables are a great source of magnesium. Magnesium is used by the body for everything it does, and all energy cells (ATP) need magnesium attached to them to work. So in these stressful, busy and important lives that we lead, extra greens won't do you any harm! Fill up on spring greens, mustard greens, kale, beetroot leaves, cabbage, dandelion, spinach, rocket, watercress, etc.

Dandelion: The roots and leaves of this plant are a great source of vitamin A and have been used in traditional medical systems to cure various health ailments, including kidney disease. Dandelion has diuretic properties, which is why it is a good tonic for the kidneys.

Parsley juice: Parsley is a diuretic and is commonly recommended for the treatment of kidney conditions. It contains not only vitamin A but also vitamin B, thiamin, riboflavin, potassium and copper. Simply chop up the parsley, boil it in water and drink it when it has cooled. Whether you have kidney problems or not, this will help flush out toxins and slow down any degenerative issues in the kidneys.

Food rich in B6: Vitamin B6 insufficiency is associated with kidney stones, so eat B6-rich foods such as avocados, sweet potatoes, cauli-flower, fish, whole grains and legumes.

Extra virgin olive oil: This oil can be used in many different recipes and can replace almost all of the other oils you use for most prepa-rations. Extra virgin olive oil is well known for its powers to soothe inflammation and detoxify the body. Therefore, it is ideal for slowing down the progression of kidney disease.

<u>Action:</u> If you find drinking water hard, here are some tips to help make you fall in love with the good stuff.

- Make a daily chart with eight pictures of water. Colour each glass in as you drink them!
- Put an alarm on your phone every hour for five hours to prompt you to take in some water – this can be anything from a large mouthful to a 225ml (8fl oz) glass, depending on where you are starting from.
- Buy a glass water bottle – try www.kleankanteen.co.uk
- Buy a water filter – try www.nikken.com

The physical body

The adrenal glands

Your adrenal glands sit on top of your kidneys, secreting cortisol in response to stress and energy requirements. So, for example, if some-one scares you, a lot can be secreted; equally, if you are about to have an appraisal by your boss or an audition or interview your cortisol levels can rise. When stress levels are high for long periods of time, physical manifestations of the physical body can arise, including premature greying of hair, excessive craving of salty foods, low libido, lower back pain, sore knees and UTI infections.

Anaemia and immune deficiency can be related to weak kidney energy as the kidneys control the growth and development of bones, the source of red and white blood cells. In traditional Chinese medicine the spinal cord and the brain are seen as forms of marrow, and therefore poor memory, the inability to think clearly and back-ache are all regarded as indicators of impaired kidney function and deficient kidney energy.

Action: Keeping your feet flat, stomp them slowly for about five minutes each day. This stimulates your kidneys' energy, as the feet are associated with the kidney and bladder meridians, which run through the heel to the sole of the foot. You can also rub your ears for several minutes each day. This simple massage strengthens kidney function, as the ears are connected energetically to the kidney organ and meridian.

HOW TO KEEP YOUR KIDNEYS HAPPY

Your kidneys will love you if you keep them well hydrated all day long. They love water, herbal tea, fresh-fruit-infused water and the occasional polyphenol-rich glass of red wine to keep your microbes working for your kidneys, as well as fresh fibre (vegetables)! Your kidneys will look after you for your whole life if you keep the toxin load low and think about what you put in your body – heavily processed foods and toxins are the very substances that mean the kidneys have to work harder.

Nutritional eating plan for a healthy pair of kidneys

All the food recommended here has health benefits to support the functions of your kidneys. You do not need to eat all the meals over the course of one day but do try to add some of them into your life. I'd suggest starting by changing your breakfast or snack. Rotation of foods is key to a diverse, creative and exciting diet.

Meals and snacks	Nutrition	Benefits
On waking in the morning	Water on waking Parsley (bunch) and ½ cucumber, cold-pressed juice, squeeze of lemon and lime	Parsley is a diuretic that helps reduce the build-up of toxins in the kidneys
First meal of the day	Chia seed and oat bowl with coconut milk, raw honey, pumpkin seeds, cinnamon and blueberries	Full of antioxidants and omega oils for their anti-inflammatory properties
Snack, if desired	Avocado slices with cherry tomatoes, red onion, hemp seeds chopped with parsley	High in vitamin C and monounsaturated fats to protect your arteries
Second meal of the day	Red quinoa, with cauli-flower rice, chopped red peppers, diced courgettes, spring onions, garlic sesame seeds and a drizzle of sesame seed oil	This dish is full of antioxidants, protein from cauliflower and quinoa. The garlic and onions have cleansing and healing properties
Snack	Lemon and garlic hummus with courgette sticks	Hummus contains good protein and fat, keeping you satisfied, as well as fresh fibre from the courgettes
Third meal of the day	Baked sea bass with sumac and spice, red lentil salad with chopped parsley and finely chopped leeks	Sumac makes this dish alive with its tangy lemon aromas: full of lean protein and healing vegetables and medicinal herbs
Bedtime snack	Dandelion leaf tea	Promotes waste and elimination

SIGNS THAT YOUR KIDNEYS ARE UNDER STRESS OR UNHAPPY

Protein in the urine: Leaking protein into the urine is not a good sign for the kidneys, but it is not a stand-alone marker of kidney failure. However, over-exercise, emotional stress, fever and extreme cold temperatures can cause a temporary elevation in protein levels in the urine.

Dark urine: This is a sign that you are not drinking enough water and you are dehydrated. If you remember nothing else, remember that the kidneys need water and long-term dehydration can cause kidney stones, which some people have attested is more painful than childbirth.[1] So drink more water – your urine should appear almost transparent.

Here are my water rules:

- Drink on waking – 250ml (9fl oz)
- Drink 10 minutes before every main meal – 250ml (9fl oz).
- Drink after every bowel movement – 250ml (9fl oz).
- Sip water also throughout the day as you desire.
- Aim to get the majority of your water intake for the day (2 litres/3½ pints) in by 6pm, because then the body starts winding down and needs less.
- If you are exercising, be mindful that you will need more water.

Lower back pain: This pain can spread down below the kidneys to your groin and between your thighs. Sometimes the pain can come and go, often in varying intensities.

Frequent urination: If you are properly hydrated, you might expect to urinate every three hours, but when your kidneys are out of balance you can urinate much more frequently. If this becomes a regular problem, it could be a sign of diabetes.

Frequent urinary tract infection: There are several reasons why people develop UTIs, but often it is because of a build-up of bacteria (the most common of which is E. coli, often found in the GIT. Women tend to suffer with UTIs more than men because the distance between the urethra and the anus and the urethral opening and the bladder is shorter, which means it's more likely for the bacteria to be moved there either through sexual intercourse or through wiping ineffectively after going to the toilet.

Abnormal urine: Abnormal urine can be brown, pink, cloudy, bloody or foul-smelling. There can also be an urge to urinate but when you do, not much empties. Foamy urine can be a sign that there is protein in the urine and should be checked with your doctor.

Ammonia breath and metallic taste: When the kidneys are not functioning properly the levels of urea in the blood (uraemia) rise. This urea is broken down into ammonia in the saliva, causing urine-smelling bad breath called ammonia breath. It is also often overlooked as a symptom associated with the kidneys.

Horsetail for the kidneys

The Roman physician Galen recommended horsetail (*Equisetum arvense*) as a treatment, and it has since been recommended as a folk remedy for kidney and bladder troubles, arthritis, bleeding ulcers and tuberculosis.

Horsetail is an astringent herb and has a diuretic action. It can be used to soothe the urinary tract of inflammation and cystitis and can also be used to assist in dissolving kidney stones.

Case study

Pub quiz

Darren was a kind man, he was someone who gave more than he took, but there was something I couldn't put my finger on when I met him with my sister last Christmas. Clare and I had snuck off to the local pub for a gin or two on Christmas Eve, and there we met Darren. There was a pub quiz in motion, so the three of us, like naughty school kids, misbehaved at the back, smugly answering questions.

Darren smoked and he drank – no great crimes – physically he was strong and mentally he was smart and astute, and yet it was as if a dark shadow had been cast over him. Emotionally I had a thought that something wasn't quite right, as a darkened facial hue can mean the kidneys are weak or out of balance. I thought it could be a kidney issue. Over the months on my trips to Somerset we got to know each other and over a cup of tea and a slice of carrot cake a few months later he told me he had only one kidney.

Most people who are born without a kidney (or with only one working kidney) lead normal, healthy lives. Sometimes people have a kidney removed during an operation in order to treat an injury or a disease like cancer, or perhaps donated a kidney to someone who needed a transplant. The strange thing about Darren was that he only found out two and a half years before – and he was 45 years old! He had not had a nephrectomy (the surgical removal of a kidney), but had a condition called renal dysplasia. So how had he got so far with one kidney? Because people can, and do, live perfectly happy lives with one kidney, the workhorses of the body.

PATHOLOGIES OF THE KIDNEYS

Kidney stones (Renal calculi)

Kidney stones are very common, and when they pass through the ureter (the tube connecting the kidneys to the bladder) they can cause severe pain in your back and sides.

Various wastes are excreted in the urine and when the toxic load in the urine increases, crystals form in the kidneys. The crystals attract more waste products then turn solid, and can get larger. Smaller stones can pass out naturally with good hydration levels but sometimes they can block the urethra when trying to exit. Think about what an amethyst crystal stone looks like – that is what your body has to pass when you have a kidney stone. In cases where stones are too large to pass, treatments may be given to remove the stones or break them down into smaller pieces which can pass out of the body.

There are many possible causes of kidney stones, including an inherited disorder that manifests in too much calcium being absorbed from foods.

Sometimes medications can help to prevent recurrent stone formation, but the best preventative measures are through your diet.

Types of stones
Uric acid stones: The main reason these are present is due to not enough fluids in the body, or because someone loses a lot of fluids or has a diet high in protein that is not being metabolised. If you suffer from gout you are also at risk of developing stones. There is reason to believe there may be a genetic factor involved in the development of these types of stones.

Calcium oxalate stones: The majority of stones found are reported to be calcium stones. They are formed of calcium oxalate, which is found in food, so it is believed that foods high in oxalate levels may contribute to kidney stones. High levels of calcium in the body also contribute, which can arise from oxalate in the liver, high vitamin D levels, metabolic disorders and calcium levels in the urine.

Struvite stones: These are present in a response to an infection, such as a urinary tract infection.

Cystine stones: These are the genetic stones found in people who excrete too much of the amino acid cystinuria.

Reasons why kidney stones may occur and what it looks or feels like for you

Most of the time the stones will pass in the urine, causing you no pain at all; however, this is not always the case. If you notice you have kidney stones and do not do something about them you will experience terrible pain that will get worse the longer you leave it. So it is worth being aware of the following signs and symptoms. It is also good to remember that if you do get stones and don't change your diet and lifestyle you will get them again, as the pathway has been created for them to take up residency in your body unless you make the necessary changes.

Blood in the urine (haematuria): Blood in the urine is not necessarily visible to the naked eye but it can be detected in a urine test or under a microscope (blood cells). Any discoloration of the urine may very well be a kidney stone and will need to be attended to with urgency. Blood in the urine is not normal.

Urinary tract infections: If you are continually experiencing infections it is likely that the root cause is not an infection but a kidney stone, so the remedy you are using will not be working well enough.

The primary cause of UTIs is condensed urine, so drink lots of water to flush away the toxins.

Dehydration: It sounds too good to be true, but the major cause of kidney stones is simply not drinking enough water. The new guidelines to prevent kidney stones recommend you drink enough water to pass 2 litres (3½ pints) of fluid every day.

Gout: If you are a male and over 40 you are in a risk group for gout and kidney stones. Gout is a build-up of uric acid in the blood and you will know you have this as your big toe will be excruciatingly painful.

Flank pain: Kidney stones or another kidney problem may also cause persistent flank pain. Although this is often a symptom of a kidney problem, it can also be the result of other medical conditions if it occurs along with additional symptoms. It's important to see your doctor if you have chronic or severe flank pain, especially if you're also experiencing other symptoms.

Other ways to help yourself through kidney stones

Avoid high-purine foods: If you are prone to developing kidney stones, cut down on high-purine foods such as red meat, organ meats and shellfish and follow a diet that contains mostly vegetables and fruits, whole grains and low-purine meats. Eating fewer animal-based proteins and more fruits and vegetables will help decrease urine acidity, and this will help reduce the chance of stone formation.

Limit sugar-sweetened foods and drinks: Especially those that contain high-fructose corn syrup.

Reduce alcohol intake: Limit alcohol because it can increase uric acid levels in the blood, and avoid crash diets for the same reason.

Action: To make life easier, have a list on your fridge of foods that strengthen your kidneys and foods that weaken them. For example:

Foods rich in magnesium:

- Dark leafy greens/whole grains/dried apricots/avocados/nuts/dark chocolate (90 per cent cocoa solids)
- Seeds/legumes

Bad foods:

- Refined sugars
- Processed meats
- Processed dairy products
- Conventional meats and products (non-organic)
- Farmed fish

Don't overdo exercise: While sweating is essential for many reasons, watch out for staying too long in saunas, hot yoga studios and heavy HIIT exercise or spin classes – overdoing exercise and sweating, especially if you are not properly rehydrating yourself, can contribute to kidney stones. Remember, the more you sweat, the less you urinate, which allows for stone-causing minerals to settle and bond in the kidneys and urinary tract. If you are urinating a lot, this is good, providing you don't have diabetes (a common symptom is frequent urination).

The three-day kidney cleanse

The aim of this cleanse is to reduce acid build-up in the kidneys and to dissolve kidney stones. Most people focus on the liver as the organ that needs cleansing and they forget about all the hard work and filtering that the kidneys must do. And while a liver cleanse is essential for good health and maintenance of the body, if you have ever suffered from a urinary infection, fluid retention or kidney stones you should consider a kidney cleanse but discuss it with your health practitioner first, particularly if you have a health problem, an eating disorder or you're pregnant.

Time	Food/herb
Upon waking	Warm water with ½ squeezed lemon 1 level teaspoon marshmallow root* in 250ml (9fl oz) hot water, the juice of ½ lemon and 1 teaspoon raw honey to sweeten
9am	Cold-pressed juice 1 (see below)
Midday	Garlic drink: crush 4 garlic cloves in 330ml (11fl oz) warm water
2pm	Cold-pressed juice 2 (see below)
4pm	1 level teaspoon marshmallow* in 250ml (9fl oz) hot water, the juice of ½ lemon and 1 teaspoon raw honey to sweeten
6pm	Cold-pressed juice 1 (see below)
Before bedtime	Power broth (see below)

* Marshmallow is a herb that helps reduce the build-up of minerals and toxins that can be stored in the bladder and kidneys. Due to its diuretic properties you may find that you urinate more, which flushes out these organs.

Cold-pressed juice 1: 8 x carrots, 1 x grapefruit, 1 x thumbnail of ginger root and 6 x celery sticks.

Cold-pressed juice 2: 1 x cucumber, 1 x medium beetroot, 1 x thumbnail of root ginger, 6 x celery sticks, 1 x small knob of turmeric and ½ squeezed lemon.

Power broth: 24-hour bone broth – chicken or beef bones. (See page 81.)

Drink nettle tea, dandelion tea or burdock tea as freely as you want over the three days.

For up to three days, depending on how you are feeling and what you are trying to achieve, follow the plan, then after the third day follow the instructions below. This is a great way to reduce water retention and cellulite as well as dissolve potential kidney stones. You can easily just do one day, as if you are not used to any drinking liquids this can be difficult.

For the next two to three days

Breakfast: Smoothie with one handful of cherries, one handful of blueberries and one handful of cranberries, along with some protein powder (for vegans, try The Beauty Chef) or gelatin powder (Great Lakes) and coconut milk or water. You can add one teaspoon of green powder, spirulina or chlorella too, if you like.

Nettle tea/dandelion tea: Loose herbs with boiling water.

Lunch: Consume another smoothie or juice similar to the one you had for breakfast.

Dinner: Eat a big salad, with green leaves and raw vegetables and a grilled chicken breast, olive oil and garden herbs to taste.

Before bed: Power tonic – one dessertspoon of gelatin with freshly chopped ginger and turmeric roots, ½ teaspoon of coconut oil, a squeeze of lemon and hot water.

Kidney cleanse herbs: To be consumed freely as a tea valerian: skullcap, wild yam, khella, marshmallow, slippery elm.

Urinary tract infections

Urinary tract infections (UTIs) occur when germs enter the urinary tract and cause symptoms such as pain and/or burning during urination and a more frequent need to urinate. These infections most often affect the bladder, but they sometimes spread to the kidneys and can cause fever and pain in your back.

Although UTIs are common and frequent occurrences, many of them are preventable with a few lifestyle changes.

Different types of infections

Cystitis: An infection of the bladder caused by the bacteria E. coli, but not exclusively. It often affects women more than men because the distance from the urethra to the anus and the urethral opening to the bladder is short.

Urethritis: Infection of the urethra when the bacteria has spread from the anus to the urethra. Sexually transmitted diseases can also cause urethritis, such as herpes, gonorrhea, chlamydia and mycoplasma.

Ureteritis: An infection of the ureter.

Pyelonephritis: An infection of the kidneys, such as E. coli.

What urinary tract infections may look or feel like for you

A burning sensation when urinating: You may feel this just before you pee and find it difficult to actually pee because of the pain.

A feeling of urgency or the need to urinate frequently: This would be abnormal to your daily urination habits. If you feel that you are getting up to pee more frequently, something needs to be addressed.

An altered appearance of the urine: A slight hint of blood or urine that is cloudy or foamy are signs you should not ignore.

Lower back pain: This is where your kidneys live, so if drinking more water does not release the pain there may be an infection, which is easy to get seen to and corrected.

How to prevent a urinary tract infection

A urinary tract infection happens in one of two ways: when outside bacteria get pushed into the urethra, or when bacteria already in the bladder multiply to unhealthy levels. Most UTIs are caused by bacteria that are already in the bladder, so flushing them out is the most important way to stave off infection.

Prevention	Why
Drink 2 litres (3½ pints) of water every day	Fluid helps move things through the urinary tract, but it also dilutes the urine so that bacteria can't grow.
Don't hold a wee for fear of missing out	As urine sits in your bladder it starts to become stagnant, like pond water, which is an ideal environment for an infection to develop in.
Women wipe from front to back	A bacterium that finds its way into your urethra comes from two places: your vagina or your rectum. Wiping back to front, especially after a bowel movement, is the main cause for rectal bacteria being introduced into the vagina and urethra.
Empty your bladder after sexual intercourse	Urinating after sex flushes out any bacteria that could have migrated to the bladder during intercourse.

Do not use perfumed products on your genitals	Douching washes out both good and bad bacteria, disrupting the natural balance of the vagina, which in turn allows bad bacteria to grow. The lactobacillus (good bacteria) in the vagina kill off bacteria that can cause UTIs. And since the vagina and the urethra sit next to each other, you want lactobacillus there to control the growth of bad bacteria. For prevention of post-intercourse UTIs, take 1 tablespoon of lactobacillus one hour prior to intercourse and another tablespoon immediately afterwards.
Take probiotics	Fermented drinks such as kombucha, fermented cabbage such as kimchi and sauerkraut and probiotic-heavy yoghurts such as kefir might help more than your digestion. Eating probiotic foods can help populate good vaginal bacteria.
Take D-mannose	Take 1 teaspoon D-mannose (about 2g) for adults, ½–1 teaspoon for children, dissolved in a glass of water and repeat every two to three hours. Continue for two to three days after symptoms have disappeared. For preventing recurring infections, start with the dosages listed above, then gradually reduce the dose, if possible. This treatment was used by Dr Jonathan Wright 20 years ago, who found the treatment to be 90 per cent effective.[2] If you suffer from frequent UTIs, it is good to have D-mannose, a kind of sugar that is related to glucose, in your holistic health cupboard.
Cranberries	Proanthocyanidins (the active ingredient in cranberries) supposedly interferes with the way that *E. coli* sticks to the wall of the bladder. Drinking cranberry juice or taking it in tablet form may help improve symptoms but there is no evidence that it will cure an infection.

Functional diagnostic testing of your kidneys

Early detection and treatment of chronic kidney disease are key to preventing kidney disease progressing to kidney failure. Some simple tests can be done to detect early kidney disease. They are:

Albumin to creatinine ratio (ACR): This estimates the amount of albumin that is in your urine. An excess amount of protein in your urine may mean your kidneys' filtering units have been damaged by disease. One positive result could be due to fever or heavy exercise, so your doctor will want to repeat this test over several weeks.

Blood creatine: Your doctor should use your results, along with your age, race, gender and other factors, to calculate your glomerular filtration rate (GFR). Your GFR tells you how much kidney function you have.

It is especially important that people who have an increased risk of chronic kidney disease have these tests. You may have an increased risk of kidney disease if your glomerular filtration rate is 90 or lower. The lower the rate, the higher the risk of full loss of kidney function.

WATER: THE MOST UNDERRATED HEALTH SOLUTION IN THE WORLD!

You might have experienced a dull pain in your back from time to time which may feel muscular and internal – that's the kidneys' way of telling you they need hydrating. Otherwise they are pretty robust and efficient and will get on with the job in hand of filtering your blood.

The body is made up of 70 per cent water and without it many processes and chemical reactions in the body could not happen. If you don't like drinking water, you are not alone. It often feels like I am asking one of the hardest things when I ask clients to drink water. The aversion to water is becoming one of epic proportions, no wonder everyone is constipated! My generation seems to like the stuff but it is the war babies who seem to dislike it most. I was in Cornwall this year at my father's 70th birthday, and as head chef I was privy to the dietary requests of the guests – there were none! The only thing they seemed to want at regular intervals throughout the day were English breakfast tea and wine – red wine for the men and white wine for the ladies. You may laugh but I'm not joking, very little other liquid passed their lips. There was, of course, the cold-pressed juice I made in the morning, which only started to be enjoyed with the addition of pear, and with that I accepted defeat and gave them what they wanted, not what I wanted to give them. I did, however, fool my mother into eating coconut oil. In the supermarket three months later, I put some coconut oil in the trolley. 'Oh no,' mother declared, 'not that awful stuff, Hannah, I really can't stand it.' 'Strange,' I said, 'in Cornwall it was the only oil you ate for the week.' In the trolley it stayed. Sometimes, just like the foods we crave are bad for us, the foods we don't like are good for us. Sorry, Mum!

The substance that was so clearly lacking that week in Cornwall was water, which is the most vital medicine for the kidneys, and drinking it is possibly the easiest thing we can do for good health. At home, not too long ago, I gave my parents a water test. I wrote our names on three 1.5-litre bottles of water and gave one to each of us, then told them they could only drink from their own bottle to see how much they drank over the course of the day. (They love it when I come home! I know I am a nag but it's only because I love them.) So the next morning when the experiment was over, Dad had consumed less than 500ml (17fl oz) of water and Mum probably just 1 litre (1¾ pints), but she did have a coughing fit that night which prompted her to down two glasses, so I'm not sure that is a fair reflection of her actual daily habits. However, she took the prize. The experiment was a revelation for them, and since then they have both improved and tell me proudly that they now start the day with a glass when they wake up. Mum often says that she drinks more than Dad, and Dad often says the same of Mum!

If you are a reluctant water drinker, try to work in some of the following suggestions and you may just start to feel better.

How to get more water into your life

When	Why
Drink water on waking	You have been asleep for 8 hours and will be dehydrated on waking
Drink after caffeine	Caffeine is a stimulant and dehydrates you if you are not already properly hydrated
Drink herbal tea	Water in disguise!
Drink water after every bowel movement	With every bowel movement you take water out of the body, so make sure to replenish it
Drink a glass of water before each meal and not with each meal	Drinking water when you eat interferes with the process of digestion and depletes the efficiency of the digestive enzymes

TOP 10 TIPS FOR HEALTHY KIDNEYS

1. **Reduce your refined sugar intake:** Eliminating sugar from your diet or reducing your sugar intake can reduce your risk of diabetes, obesity and kidney disease. If you cut back on processed sugars you're also likely to reduce your intake of calories, chemicals and sodium. Your kidneys and your waistline will thank you!

2. **Keep your blood pressure in check:** If you have high blood pressure your heart will have to work harder to pump blood and oxygen around the body. In some cases high blood pressure can lead to heart attacks, strokes and organ failure, including of your kidneys.

3. **Keep your weight in check:** Excess body fat can adversely affect the health of your kidneys while some dietary fat may be beneficial. The

more fat you have around your kidneys, the greater your chances of developing kidney disease, especially if you have type 2 diabetes.

4. **Snack on cranberries:** Not only can these little berries help with symptoms of urinary tract infections but they also help the prevention of kidney stone formation. Cranberries contain antibacterial compounds known as tannins, which prevent bacteria sticking to the walls of the bladder and the kidneys.

5. **Eat red peppers:** High in vitamin C and antioxidants, as well as helping to rid the body of free radicals and inflammations. The red pepper has an effect on stimulating the secretion of saliva and gastric juice, which improves appetite. It is also a food low in potassium, is sweet and full of flavour, all of which makes it a great food for the kidneys.

6. **Eat kale:** Kale is one of the most versatile vegetables if you start thinking outside of the box. You can steam it, bake it and flavour it into chips, add it to casseroles or raw to a salad. It is another vegetable that is low in potassium and high in iron, which you may be lacking if you have a kidney problem. It's also an all-round immunity booster and anti-inflammatory food.

7. **Grapefruit for breakfast:** Apart from being a great source of vitamin C, grapefruit is also very low in potassium, which makes it a friend of the kidneys.

8. **Decrease your sodium intake:** Large quantities of sodium can increase blood pressure levels. High blood pressure damages the kidneys over time and is a leading cause of kidney failure. Instead, use Himalayan or Celtic sea salt to flavour and season your food.

9. **Drink filtered water:** Your kidneys need water to help the body wash out all the waste and your blood needs replacement water all the time.

10. **Juice and drink celery:** The coumarins in celery help clear metabolic waste products, which are byproducts that get sent to the lymphatic system then to the kidneys for removal via urine.

Footnotes

(1) Lindsay, D., '13 Agonising pains that are worse that child-birth – according to mums and scientists', metro.co.uk/201 6/08/24/13-agonising-pains-that-are-worse-than-childbirth -according-to-mums-and-scientists-6087726/ (accessed on 05/01/2018).

(2) Wright, Dr J. V., 'D-Mannose for Bladder and Kidney Infections', *Natural Medicine Articles* (Tahoma, 2011).

5. THE PANCREAS

A sweetness of life

The pancreas releases hormones into the blood to control blood sugars (glucose), so when you eat sugar the pancreas responds by releasing a hormone called insulin. If you keep feeding your body sugar, often in the form of abundant carbohydrates such as sweets, chocolate, cakes, fizzy drinks, refined sugar, alcohol or fruit, insulin is consistently released in an attempt to control your blood glucose levels. It's really that simple, but resources, like hormones, have a habit of running out or running dry, and insulin and glucagon are no exception to this rule.

Sugar lurks in every shop corner, on every restaurant's dessert trolley and it lingers in everyone's mind. Just think how easily Willy Wonka was able to seduce those unlikeable children into his factory and expose their addictive traits and beastly personalities with the drug we know so well – sugar. Just because you don't eat gummy bears or jelly sweets, that doesn't exempt you from being a sugar addict. Sugar is a bit of a monster for the pancreas; it sits on your shoulder and constantly nudges you to make the wrong decisions; it has its claws into many of us and has such a hold that most of us struggle dreadfully to get rid of it.

If you are unable to take control of your sugar addiction you may start to experience some rather inconvenient signs, such as frequent urination or constant thirst, both of which are caused when your insulin is running low or running out. The pancreas naturally resists change, so if you do have a sugar problem you'll have to dig deep to make those changes, but this is well within your grasp and you will feel better for it in the long run.

> **Facts:**
>
> ● The pancreas releases hormones into the blood to control blood sugars (glucose).
> ● A discoloration of the bridge of the nose can signal blood-sugar handling problems.
> ● Many parts of the world eat the pancreas of various animals, and it is considered a very rich food.
> ● The pancreas is roughly 12.5 centimetres (5 inches) long.

A BIT MORE ANATOMY

The pancreas is a multifunctional organ and leaf-shaped gland without ducts that lies posteriorly and slightly below the borders of the stomach and the walls of the duodenum. The pancreas has two major jobs:

1. **Secretion of digestive juices which aid digestion.** The exocrine cells of the pancreas are tasked with developing these enzymes, which are released when food enters the stomach, and aid digestion of fats, carbohydrates and proteins in the food that you eat in the duodenum (the first part of the small intestine). The digestive juices are alkaline and so neutralise the acids that creep through from the stomach, thus creating an optimal environment in which the enzymes can work.

2. **Production of hormones to regulate blood glucose levels.** The pancreas has a head, a tail and a body, with each cell producing the hormones insulin and glucagon. Insulin has the function of

lowering the level of blood glucose while glucagon increases it, and they work together to maintain the right balance of glucose (sugar) in the blood.

The health of the pancreas requires a fully functional stomach, spleen, liver and gallbladder. It is more and more common to see pancreatic insufficiency these days; the root of digestive complaints is modern fast-paced lifestyles and convenience food that is eaten in a rush without any thought given to what you are eating. The cephalic phase of gastric secretion occurs even before food enters the stomach, especially while it is being chewed in the mouth. It results from the sight, smell, thought or taste of food, and the greater the appetite, the more intense the stimulation. Without a cephalic response, digestion will be impaired. My first prescription for clients complaining of digestive issues is to take 30–60 minutes for lunch and eat with a friend, walk to get your lunch or take a stroll after lunch and do not dine with your computer or phone. The latter is usually the most difficult for people to conquer, as taking a picture of your food for social media seems to be protocol these days!

Did you know?

One of the most unique functions of the pancreas is that it creates bicarbonate, which is similar to the bicarbonate of soda that your mum might have advised you to take when you have an upset stomach from time to time. It has a neutralising effect on the stomach's acidic environment which assists digestion.

ENERGIES OF THE PANCREAS

The meridian of the pancreas

The meridian of the pancreas shares the same meridian as the spleen and begins on the middle border of the big toe, ascends through the leg, thigh, abdomen and lateral border of the ribcage and drops down to the axilla (inner legs, groin and ribs).

The pancreas meridian affects the spleen, pancreas, menstruation, adrenals, groin area and organs, lower diaphragm and sense of taste. When it is out of balance one can experience gastritis, indigestion, abdominal distention, ulcers, vomiting, pain in the lower extremities, irregular menstrual cycle, anaemia and generally being run down.

Properties of the pancreas meridian

Force: Yin (female)

Chakra: Solar plexus – personal power, self-will

Organ body clock: 9–11am

Season: Summer (Indian)

Colours: Orange and yellow

Fragrances: Sweet and minty

Metaphysical lesson: Reflection and sympathy (overly abundant or lack of)

Emotions of the pancreas

Energetically, the pancreas allows love and gratitude into our lives, controlling the flow of sweetness. If the pancreas is weak you may be struggling to receive love, and when a person cannot accept love they grow bitter over time and may feel that they are missing out on life or that life is passing them by. By practising gratitude you can heal any feelings of bitterness and therefore allow sweetness to flow into your life. The pancreas is located in the third chakra, an accessory organ to the digestive system. It is often referred to as the seat of your emotional life, as it is where your personal power comes from. Here your sensitivity, ambition and ability to achieve are stored. If there is a blockage in the third chakra the pancreas may be out of balance; your sugar cravings may increase but you may also lose your personal power and become frustrated with your choices and your life.

THE FOUR BODIES OF THE PANCREAS

The spiritual body

We can only postulate on the mind–body emotional connection to a diseased organ, but specifically with the pancreas you can find parallels that simulate our behaviours and our life. If the pancreas represents a sweetness of life and disease represents a long-standing hurt and resentment, the parallels between nutrition, emotion and the spiritual body are apparent. If you turn it around and say that not being able to find a sweetness of life is similar to grief because you are holding on, you are also not digesting life and will have an inability to break it down, which is one of the functions of the pancreas. When we are overcome with anxiety, we block our ability to heal as well as access to our resources to be able to think clearly and to be positive. Stress and unpleasant situations will always occur, but it is how we deal with them and the overview that we have of them that make the sweetness of life flow.

Action: Guided meditation is a great way to start to make some positive changes in your life that will allow you to seek out what you want and how you want things to be in your life.

The emotional body

The pancreas is a reservoir of energy and is associated with the third chakra, which is associated with our own personal power. It is where we learn to have a strong sense of ourselves and where we come into our own. When the third chakra is weak we lead from a place of insecurity and we put our ego in charge. Chronic feelings of despair, anguish and hopelessness are the cause of a pancreas being out of balance, and when someone loses the sweetness of life and becomes burdened with its struggle, through self-bitterness, self-rejection and self-hatred, it is not uncommon for diabetes to surface.

The pancreas is an organ of stability and so it will resist change. It is in charge of maintaining the primary source of energy in the body and its purpose is survival, so any changes that challenge this purpose can be greeted with resistance.

The pancreas is affected by the disappointment of other people's decisions. The lesson here is about learning to accept situations without any expectations. This is one of the hardest lessons, but when you master it you see most situations and opportunities as a gift and you begin to see the sweetness of life and don't dwell on what you don't have, instead feeling an abundance of joy.

Action: Go into each situation without any expectation, then you can only be pleasantly surprised, not disappointed. Next time you go to a restaurant or meet a friend, go to the cinema or the theatre, go with an open mind. Maybe don't read too many reviews, or listen to too many opinions, then you will have space to make up your own mind.

The nutritional body

Regular consumption of refined-sugar goods, processed foods, caffeine and alcohol are all very damaging as they will overstimulate the production of insulin and weaken the pancreas over time.

Action: Reduce your intake of refined-sugar goods, processed honey and commercial fruit juices as well as processed meats and baked goods. Chew food thoroughly and slow the eating process by putting the fork down routinely throughout the meal for optimum digestion. Favour wholesome unprocessed foods such as whole grains, vegetables and pulses. Avoid having more than four hours without food; if you do require snacks, there are a few ideas below.

Avocado dip: Blend 1 avocado with 1 teaspoon of chilli, paprika, a pinch of sea salt and a squeeze of lime.

Dip in raw vegetable soldiers (e.g. carrot, courgette, cucumber, peppers).

Bean and mint dip: Empty a can of chickpeas into a blender with 3 tablespoons of olive oil, 1 tablespoon of garlic-infused oil or 3 crushed cloves and a handful of mint leaves.

Dip in raw vegetable soldiers (e.g. carrot, courgette, cucumber, peppers).

Red pepper, cherry tomato and basil soup: Roast a red pepper and blend with 5 cherry tomatoes, black pepper, sea salt, crushed garlic and fresh basil leaves.

Dip in raw vegetable soldiers (e.g. carrot, courgette, cucumber, peppers).

Pea or broad bean and mint dip: Pour 150g (5 oz) of garden peas into a blender with 3 tablespoons of olive oil and a handful of mint leaves, and blend.

Dip in raw vegetable soldiers (e.g. carrot, courgette, cucumber, peppers).

The physical body

The physical signs of the pancreas being out of balance – besides cravings for sugar and carbohydrates – are overeating and eating too quickly, feeling frequently thirsty or sleepy after eating and drinking alcohol, bruising easily, being sensitive to strong smells, having a craving for processed foods, digestive discomfort and flatulence that is not immediately linked to eating (i.e. appearing 2–3 hours after eating), waking in the middle of the night but feeling sleepy during the day.

Action: You can support the pancreas by doing breathing exercises to help yourself relax, or singing to reduce anxiety and to help express yourself. Getting out of your comfort zone by socialising with others and doing charitable deeds will help redress the emotional imbalances within this organ.

HOW TO LOOK AFTER YOUR PANCREAS

Your pancreas will love you if you keep excitement and adventure in your life. Always have something to look forward to, like a holiday, a massage or a day off seeing something new. The pancreas loves brightly coloured foods that come from this earth, and these will help keep it balanced, physically and emotionally. The pancreas loves receiving small amounts of food regularly throughout the day and not a lot of food at once. So be kind to your pancreas by taking the time to eat your homemade, brightly coloured seasonal creations.

Nutritional plan for a healthy pancreas

Meals and snacks	Nutrition	Benefits
On waking in the morning	Filtered water	Hydration
First meal of the day	**Spicy eggs:** Eggs x 2 with ½ diced red pepper, ½ courgette and ¼ red onion, fry with coconut oil and season with sea salt, black pepper, turmeric, paprika, chilli and cayenne pepper	Spice for a speedy metabolism
Snack, if desired	**Cucumber canapés:** Chop medium cucumber slices and top with hummus, olive tapenade, feta, basil and sun-dried tomatoes	Easy to digest foods with all three macronutrients
Second meal of the day	**Tossed tuna:** Tuna steak seared on a low heat, served on a bed of tossed rocket and watercress, Tenderstem broccoli and pine nuts	Protein and omega 3 to reduce inflammation and greens for magnesium to help relax the digestive system
Snack	Green apple	To regulate blood glucose levels
Third meal of the day	Grilled minute steak with lamb's lettuce, washed and tossed with green beans, radishes and artichoke hearts	Good saturated fats in the steak will make you feel satisfied and lean
Bedtime snack / activity	Honey, lemon and ginger tea	Helps curb sugar cravings

SIGNS THAT YOUR PANCREAS IS UNDER STRESS OR UNHAPPY

Pain in the upper abdomen: The pancreas lies just behind your stomach at the back of the body. The pain usually occurs in the upper abdomen and can radiate, feeling like back pain; it may come and go and the level can fluctuate – it might be more severe after eating, drinking alcohol or while lying down.

Bloating: The pancreas is responsible for releasing digestive enzymes (elastase) and when they are in short supply you may feel bloated or full, especially after eating, as the food is not being broken down as well as it might.

Loss of appetite and weight loss: This is due to malabsorption of food. You can eat the finest food and take the finest supplements, but if your body does not absorb them you are not receiving energy from them.

SUGAR AND THE PANCREAS

Why do all the bad things taste so good?

If there is a new swear word on the street, it goes by the name of sugar. I see people's faces change when the word is nervously muttered. Everyone claims not to eat it or not to have touched it for years and they wax lyrical about how much better their life is without it.

Sugar has become the forbidden drug of the twenty-first century. But what is sugar and where does it hide and why is it in your diet? All good questions that I am going to explain in the simplest way I know, so that it resonates, makes sense and, ultimately, so that you can decide what you want to change if you feel you need to do so.

Change is always in our hands, but we often don't make the change that is needed, because committing ourselves to big changes can seem too daunting, and we forget that we can make small alterations to get there. Don't wait until pain or illness, such as diabetes, forces your hand to make a change.

Where is sugar in my diet?

Sugar is the generic name for carbohydrates that taste sweet. Carbohydrates provide the body with energy. You can tell which foods are sugar because they will have 'ose' on the end of their name.

There are essentially four types of sugar:

Maltose: Found in beer and malt products.

Sucrose: More commonly known as table sugar and made up of glucose and fructose. Sucrose is predominantly extracted from sugar cane or sugar beet and will also be found in fruits and vegetables.

Lactose: This is often called 'milk sugar' and found in all dairy products.

Fructose and glucose: Found in honey and fruits and, to a lesser degree, vegetables.

Sugar is needed for the brain and the body to function[1]; 120g (4 oz) a day is needed to keep you going. However, it is worth remembering that that amount can come from vegetables alone!

Why do we crave sugar and what are your cravings telling you?
Sugar: have you really given it up?
If I had a pound for everyone who has ever said to me they have given up sugar I would most certainly be retiring on a beach in Bali. Sugar has got its claws into the best of us and, just like an obsession with

a lover or a fixation on a way of life, sugar makes us do things we wouldn't normally do and think about things we don't really want to think about. Sugar creates disharmonic harmony, but the problem is that its shelf-life is so short you keep feeding the body the drug to get the high.

Diabetes is one of the most prevalent states of disease in the Western world and it is purely down to our diets being crammed full of hidden and unhidden sugar. Couple that with our addictive traits and lack of self-control, and we are really up against it. With all that said, though, it is important to know that type 2 diabetes is both preventable and reversible.

However, there is not a pill that can reverse this health state, or a pill that will control your diabetes, the only way to reverse diabetes is to reduce your sugar intake, drop the addictions and find your self-control. This is key to preventing ill health.

Educate yourself

Tom gave up alcohol in January, along with the majority of the British population! All was going well until the food diaries started to flood in. 'What's this?' I said, pointing at one entry. 'Oh, someone's birthday at work,' he replied, 'but it was carrot cake so I thought, well, it could be worse and it's got carrot in it, so that's all good, no?'

Tom was grossly obese and fairly ignorant about food. I pointed out another entry for cheesecake. 'Did you have friends round?' 'No,' Tom replied, 'I just had one to myself.' 'One whole cheesecake? One whole cheesecake to yourself?' 'Yes, but it was only one.' He had misinterpreted, or interpreted, a treat as being a whole cake not a slice. Madness, you may think; he must be simple or stupid or playing a joke, but this story is one of hundreds of similar stories which are funny initially but underpin a huge void of education about what food is and how it creates health or disease. We regularly accept that excess alcohol can be fatal for the liver. We accept that smoking can be fatal to the lungs. However, we seem to give food a pass when it comes to disease. If your intention in January is to be alcohol-free, you may well feel smug at your success, but I bet the month wasn't sugar-free!

Take John, who decided to be virtuous and have three days a week off alcohol and drink cold-pressed juice (beetroot and apple) from a wine glass instead. On a home visit one day the fridge was stocked with cartons of apple and cranberry juice. 'What is all this?' I said. 'Juice,' said John. 'Yes, I can see it's juice but you have a cold-press juicer and you are juicing apples so why do you need the cartoned stuff as well?' 'Oh, well, it's good for me, isn't it?'

Clients often swap alcohol for fruit juice, cake for mangos and melons and pop grapes into their mouths like tennis ball servers stuck on fire. While all these changes could be argued to be a better alternative, the root cause of the underlying issue has not been addressed, just sidelined.

Perhaps it's not entirely our fault, though, because consumerism is influencing our every move. If it makes our life easier, then let's have it! Just look at where we have got to. Shouting at a small hockey puck in the middle of the room like a servant, 'Alexa, where are my socks? Alexa, where are my keys? Alexa, what's the weather doing?' I'm surprised Alexa isn't in counselling or therapy. Alexa needs to be up for the next Noble Peace Prize for the flak she takes.

So here are some alternatives that might make you think before buying the next convenient gadget; they will save you money and doing it yourself you could argue was meditation!

- Potato peeler or julienne peeler will do almost the same as a spiraliser.
- Sharpen your knives so you don't have to buy pre-chopped vegetables.
- Buy a slow cooker so your meal is ready when you get home.
- Take a month off from buying anything apart from the essentials (e.g. food) – that will empower you.
- Use a Thermos flask and always make your first coffee at home; that way you save money and the planet by not using paper coffee cups.

● Always take a banana with you to work as a snack; it gets less bounced around than other fruits without their own case.

We overconsume food and goods, then we overeat and then over-analyse what we have eaten and what we have bought. Sometimes we just need to be still, take a step back, count to 10, do three star jumps and look at the situation again.

Now, what is it that you need?

PATHOLOGIES OF THE PANCREAS

Insulin resistance and type 2 diabetes

Diabetes is a metabolic disorder characterised by a deficiency or absence of insulin due to impaired production or resistance, causing a disruption of carbohydrate and fat metabolism and elevated blood glucose levels leading to hypoglycaemia. About 90–95 per cent of people with diabetes have type 2, and although it is often found in older people, we are now seeing this proliferate among teenagers. It is also estimated that many people are pre-diabetic without knowing about it.

Types of diabetes
Type 1 diabetes: A condition where the beta cells of the pancreas make very little or no insulin and so it must be injected into the body on a regular basis to stabilise the effects of blood glucose.

Excess sugar gets stored as fat in the adipose tissues.

Type 2 diabetes: People with type 2 diabetes have an inability to utilise glucose or sugar through loss of insulin sensitivity or inability of the cell to utilise carbohydrates.

Gestational: Occurs during pregnancy as a result of placental hormones blocking insulin action in the mother. Usually disappears after delivery and returns as type 2 years later.

What type 2 diabetes might look and feel like to you

Polyuria: The need to urinate frequently. If you find yourself going to the bathroom every hour to pass small amounts of urine you might want to check your blood glucose levels with the doctor or using a monitor you can buy from a pharmacy.

Polydipsia: An increased thirst and fluid intake. If you find that you still feel thirsty when you drink water and you are drinking a lot, see the doctor.

Polyphagia: This is when your appetite has increased but nothing else in your life has changed and you are particularly seeing an increased desire for sweet foods – this may be a sign of pre-diabetes.

Glycosuria: Glucose in the urine. You can assess this on a urine screen from the doctor or a urine dip test, then you can check your sugar intake on a regular basis to see if your new diet and lifestyle changes are having an impact.

Blurred vision: This could just be temporary and is not necessarily a marker of diabetes on its own, but it can be caused by high blood sugar levels which cause the lens of the eye to swell and impairs your ability to see.

Diabetic ketoacidosis (DKA): A condition characterised by repeatedly high blood sugar levels. You can test this by peeing on a ketone stick to see the ketone levels in your urine. When the body is unable to use glucose for energy because of a lack of insulin, the body uses alternative tissue sources for energy.

Tachycardia: This is an increase in heart rate and you will find that your breath increases rapidly and deeply – it can also lend a fruity smell to your breath due to exhaled acetone. Address this immediately.

Dehydration: This will cause weakness, fatigue and mental status changes, weight loss, nausea and vomiting, blurred vision, predisposition to infections and lethargy.

How to prevent insulin resistance and diabetes

Ancel Keys did a study back in the 1950s that found the more fat eaten in a country, the greater the risk of heart disease (see page 108). Subsequently this was proven not to be true, mainly because the seven countries he chose all had high fat consumption and high heart disease levels. Since then critics have pointed out that choosing a different group of countries could produce precisely the opposite result. Secondly, this was an observational study so it didn't prove causation anyway. It did, however, prove influential because Keys was a great promoter and was ruthless about crushing and hounding his critics. One of these was John Yudkin, who wrote a book in the 1970s that pointed the finger at cane sugar. His view is now widely accepted. Counter-claim after counter-claim followed, with millions being spent on bigger studies, none of which managed to prove that a low-fat diet cut mortality rates.[2]

So today we find that dieticians and health professionals still give advice and cling to the belief that there is evidence that the low-fat diet as set out in the Eatwell Guide should form the basis of your diet. You can see a current picture of the food pyramid chart in circulation today on the NHS website.[3]

The fats that you most certainly do not want in your diet are listed below, as they are artificial and create toxicity in the body and are stored in adipose tissues, creating metabolic-type disease states such as diabetes. Most of these trans fats are hidden in our starchy carbohydrates, which is why I have added the table below to help you find them in your diet, the newsagent's or your local supermarket.

Never eat these foods	What they do	Where will I find it?
Fructose corn syrup	This is made from corn starch and is highly processed, making it toxic to the body and creating insulin resistance	In fizzy drinks, cakes, sweets, biscuits and in the majority of cheap processed foods
Trans fats	These block the flow of blood around the body, contributing to heart disease and atherosclerosis	There are two types of trans fat: naturally occurring trans fatty acids found at low levels in meat and dairy products, and artificially made trans fatty acids, labelled as hydrogenated fats or oils in some processed foods
Margarine	Margarine is a trans fat which is stored in the body's tissues as fat. It is also a hydrogenated oil that is high in omega 6 (see page 208). Use lard instead for shortening	In every sandwich or wrap you buy, and on buttered toast – it may be in your fridge. When you ask for butter, ask to see the packet so you know it's not margarine
Anything artificially coloured	Food additives change the colour of your food. Are we all, later in life, going to regret drinking the milk from our cereal that ended up a murky rainbow colour? Blue foods and drinks are full of chemicals and made in a laboratory not a kitchen	Cereals, gummy sweets, bubblegum-flavoured drinks, icing on cakes and biscuits, pastries
Processed foods	These have been altered/ injected and treated with chemicals to increase shelf life	Sliced meats and cheese. Microwave foods

Anything that goes in a microwave	Nothing nutritionally good comes out alive from a microwave, and if you have digestive issues, throw out these foods	Microwave meals, reheating food
Fizzy drinks	They are liquid sugar; they will play havoc with your blood sugar levels and weight	Cola, lemonade, everything that fizzes when you take the lid off – unless, of course, it is sparkling water

Case study

Born fit

Bill was one of the fittest 70-year-olds I have ever had the pleasure to meet, and certainly not your most likely suspect for type 2 diabetes. At 5 foot 7 and 9 stone 10 you would have thought that diabetes would have been the least of his problems.

Bill was born fit; he trained at the Nautical College, Pangbourne, before serving in the Royal Marines in his early twenties for nearly six years. After the Marines, Bill flew commercial helicopters until he was 66 years old, hanging up his flying gloves in 2010. At the age of 59, on a six-monthly aircrew medical examination by a nurse, he was declared the fittest, healthiest man she had seen for his age, strides above most 35-year-olds. It would be fair to say he led a physically active, if not strenuous, life and his vocation undoubtedly put him in heightened situations of stress.

The first sign that something wasn't quite right was during a routine check-up when his blood pressure was slightly out of range. Bill's family concurred he had a sweet tooth and I too have seen this first-hand. They told me that there were times when he would eat chocolate ice cream twice a day; however, with his level of fitness it was deemed acceptable. His doctor, whom he was very fond of, suggested a diet that essentially took away his ice cream, decreased his intake of white potatoes and all the things that cause you to want to eat more, namely starchy carbohydrates, and told him to come back in three weeks' time to have his insulin levels checked. If he was in range, he would not have to take the normally prescribed medication. Observing Bill over the week that I stayed with him, he certainly had a healthy appetite and would finish all the leftovers rather than leave them for another meal, and he was also a slow eater, which is good, but maybe that was because he was just always telling a story. If Bill had not been through all the rigorous training and exercise I wonder what his weight would be now.

Carbohydrates feed carbohydrates, and these were Bill's sweet spot. So after following the diet, his blood sugar levels regulated and he didn't have to take the medication. Things are not always what they seem; doing lots of exercise does not exempt you from following a healthy diet. Exercise does not make up for a diet high in sugar, and just because you are a healthy weight does not always mean you are healthy. Bill and his sugar cravings, addictions and self-control will always be there, but now he has had to find a way to moderate all of them.

A healthy eating plan to balance your blood sugars

It's all about balancing blood sugar levels. If you have been told that you are in the risk group for insulin resistance, have three days a week where you eat only vegetables, berries, meat, fish and eggs until your levels come down.

Time	Eat this	Instead of this
Breakfast	Dark rye/spelt/sourdough toast with olive oil, rocket and 1 poached egg	White toast with jam and a bowl of cereal with semi- skimmed cow's milk
Mid-morning snack (choose one)	Bowl of berries Apple and nut butter Dark chocolate rice cracker with Americano or herbal tea	Chocolate bar/biscuit Latte or mocha
Lunch	Baked sweet potatoes with chilli, tuna and olives or vegetable and ginger stir-fry	Pasta or pizza, or sandwich or wrap
Mid-afternoon snack	Cucumber discs with nut butter or hummus with a green tea	Latte with biscuits or slice of cake
Dinner	Salmon with avocado, broccoli and cherry tomato salad	Steak pie or an oven-baked chicken Kiev with frozen vegetables
Midnight snack	Ginger, honey, lemon	Milk chocolate

Other preventative measures for type 2 diabetes

Eat fish: It is always a good idea to have lots of fish or fish oils in your diet. Getting omega 3 fatty acids into your diet is the preferred option, especially if you have type 2 diabetes. Studies have shown that fish oil supplements may lower triglyceride levels in people with type 2 diabetes, which could also lower their risk of heart disease.

Get all three of your macronutrients: Make sure you are getting all three of your macronutrients in your diet: fat, protein and carbohydrates.

Take supplements: You can take many supplements that will help regulate blood sugar levels; some of my favourites are blue-green algae, hibiscus tea and chromium-rich foods which can help regulate blood sugar and diabetes – you can take chromium as a supplement but you will also find it naturally in broccoli.

Eat fewer grains: Decreasing your whole-grain intake will also stabilise and balance your blood sugar levels. Swap white bread for brown bread, swap brown bread for wholemeal artisan bread and then have days without grains to lower your blood glucose.

Do exercise: Being overweight is not always a marker for diabetes, but exercise can help reduce your weight and lower your sugar intake, and in turn you can make changes to your mood, body and outlook on life. Get active doing a sport or some form of exercise that you enjoy. A little trampoline in the garden is a great way to shake up the body every morning while breathing in some fresh air and stimulating your metabolism for breakfast.

Relax: Despair, anguish and hopelessness can affect the balance of your pancreas, and when you become weighed down with emotional issues for a period of time it is not uncommon for diabetes to surface. Relax your overstressed body in a bath of lavender drops and magnesium salts to reduce the anxiety and stress on your mind, soul and body. Run a bath, add the drops and the salts. Play some calming music and relax your mind.

Case study

The end of the affair

Chloe was having an affair. She had secretly entwined herself into a beautiful relationship with sugar and had become almost an expert in deception. The first time she tasted the silky-smooth sweetness of this oasis, the instant pain relief became a crutch which helped in almost any trauma in her life. Such is the nature of an affair that you make desperate or half-hearted attempts to stop because you know it's bad but somehow that makes you want it more. This affair showed no signs of ending.

When we learn traits from childhood and we only realise in adulthood they no longer work, it's an even harder job to repair the damage. I love my sugar babies (sugar addicts); they may tell you they are happy and there will be many aspects of their life they are grateful for and reasons why they should not be complaining, but essentially they are paper ships, drowning in low self-esteem. So my first challenge is to prove they are worth it; prove they are worth every penny that they are spending and that they deserve to be happy, to be thin, to wear the trousers that mark success and to feel fit, fantastic and fabulous.

'I just can't justify spending money on myself,' Chloe would say when I recommended she make appointments to see me regularly until the weight started to drop off. 'So what's expensive to you?' I asked. When you know what 'your expensive' is and when you know what you value, then you can justify the expenditure. Some people will value themselves or their health so highly that the price is not an issue, they know what they want. Part of the issue was that she was so used to spending money on her husband and her children that she had forgotten what it felt like to put herself first. She said she wouldn't have blinked at paying for her family to see me. Plus, she was having this affair, which can limit rational thought processes, self-belief and confidence, because once sugar takes up residency in someone's life it is hard to evict it.

As I presented Chloe with her wellness plan that I had written for her (see below) she said to me, 'I can't eat all that, I'll gain weight!' 'Chloe,' I answered her, 'you spend all morning with your head in the biscuit tin, trust me on this one. Like so many women wanting to lose weight, starting the day with nothing or a latte and seeing how far you can get without eating seems like a good strategy until you end up in the kitchen cupboard at 4pm or 1am stuffing cheese, hummus, baby pittas, the kids' chocolate biscuits and umpteen rice cakes with nut butter and maybe a spot of jam down your neck. It would be fair to admit the strategy needs revising. Starvation sets you up for failure – as your blood sugar levels drop you end up needing a sugar kick which spirals out of control, and trust me, you will never find any satisfaction at the bottom of a bag of sweets, just a whopping headache an hour later, maybe a bit of guilt, followed by a slap of shame and then the guaranteed sugar blues.'

Chloe's wellness plan

	Option 1:	Option 2:
Upon waking	0.5 litre (1 pint) of water	0.5 litre (1 pint) of water
Breakfast	Smoothie with berries and vegan protein powder, flaxseed oil or seeds, 1 handful of spinach, coconut water or milk	2 x poached eggs with 2 x smoked salmon slices, wilted spinach and ½ avocado
Mid-morning snack	Cold-pressed juice – 5 x carrots, thumbnail of ginger and 1 x apple	Cold-pressed juice – 5 x carrots, thumbnail of ginger and 1 x apple
Lunch	Chicken and tossed green salad	Prawn stir-fry
Mid-afternoon snack (Rule: always drink a pint of water then ask yourself if you are hungry before you eat)	2 x slices of toasted rye bread with nut butter (almond) and apple	2 x slices of sourdough bread, toasted, with goat's cheese, spinach and cucumber

Dinner	Baked fish and vegetables	Slow-cooked dishes
Before bed	Lemon + ginger tea	Lemon + ginger tea

After all, life is not about deprivation, it's about abundance.

Being healthy is about having a healthy relationship with food, which is why this book is about getting people back to the basics of how to eat, not how to make a cardboard cookie with 10 powders and super-foods in it. My job is to empower people to get back into the kitchen and start feeding themselves well and loving themselves.

Chloe was an excellent cook, so with her I just needed to reignite her fire. She was mentally ready to make the changes needed, and because she was ready she saw results and the weight just started falling off! Often I work with mothers and daughters together and the mother often exhibits the stronger mental attitude and will-power to make a start. I can see the passion and the motivation in these beautiful Boudiccas; the daughters have a much more 'laissez-faire' attitude, a sense of entitlement to their success. The message I have is that results and success always lie with you; I am just your support to help you achieve your goals. Sugar babies initially need regular support every week and then every two weeks. If you let go of their hand they no longer have the support they need.

In session two there were tears of joy from Chloe, and for me tears I fought to hold back, as with glee she couldn't believe how easy the week had been and that she was now 3kg (6½ lb) lighter and excited about food again. It was lift-off!

At session three Chloe was 4.5kg (10 lb) lighter. 'I feel well for the first time in years,' she said. She was happy to be spending the money on herself and was taking walks every day on the heath. Friends said she was glowing. At session four she told me that her friends had re-marked that she seemed happier than ever; she was 6 kilos (1 stone) lighter, calmer and sleeping better. 'This is not hard,' she said to me, almost in amazement.

When Chloe reached the 10kg (22 lb) weight-loss mark I told her to watch out for the female saboteurs. She assured me that everyone she knew was supportive and this wouldn't be a problem. However, I know it can happen; it does so all the time with females; when one leaves the pack, goes off and empowers herself, changes her lunch order, gym class or alcohol habits without the approval of the pack, they can feel ousted. I've seen women lose a huge amount of weight only to be left feeling sad that their friends are less than kind or generous about their success. Don't lose too much, don't go too far, is often the advice from the female wolf pack. Perhaps Middleton was on to something when he wrote *Women Beware Women*![4]

Today Chloe is in control and has lost a total of 12kg (1 stone 12½ lb), and in the months we worked together the pounds have never been added back. Plateauing is inevitable but that is just part of the journey – it's not just the physical body that is changing.

If you have a friend who is making the changes of a lifetime, join in the journey with her. It can take courage to do it on your own, which is why I work very closely with my clients so that I am always there when they need me. Making changes is about support. So if you have a friend who is struggling, ask her how you can help; you will make her day.

Some top tips:

- Put a chart of your plans or a calendar with your goals on the fridge for the whole family to see, then reward yourself when you get there.
- Ask your children to help you.
- Ask your family to kindly tell you off when they see you heading for the biscuit tin.
- Make an announcement on social media/a private group to rally support.

Polycystic ovaries and polycystic ovary syndrome (PCOS)

So what is polycystic ovary syndrome? It is a condition resulting from high levels of androgens (male hormones) secreted by the ovaries, namely testosterone. Having this imbalance can also mean that you may have cysts on the ovaries. Having high testosterone levels for women can mean more body and facial hair, pelvic pain, irregular periods and, ultimately, difficulty getting pregnant.

PCOS affects your hormones and your metabolism.

If you are wondering why PCOS is in the chapter on the pancreas, it is because of the hormone insulin. Insulin is produced by the pancreas and regulates, among other things, blood sugar levels. When there is an imbalance in your insulin and glucose levels you can gain weight and increase your chance of insulin resistance. This then affects your levels of oestrogen and the body's ability to clear it out of the adipose tissues, thereby increasing your risk of PCOS.

One of the most common complaints of women who present with PCOS is the almost urgent cravings for carbohydrate-based foods and sweets. The reason why women with PCOS crave more sweets than women without this condition is due to insulin, which is a powerful growth hormone that works as an appetite stimulant and causes weight gain easily, making it even more difficult to lose weight. Insulin creates a vicious cycle; when you give in to the uncontrollable sugar urge your blood sugar increases, resulting in more insulin being secreted to cope with the flood of sugar through the bloodstream. Too much sugar eaten consistently over time will end in insulin resistance and weight gain. Not only will women with PCOS struggle with insulin regulation but insulin spikes can play havoc with your blood pressure levels and cause high triglyceride levels and high levels of an inflammation marker called C-reactive protein. All these have been linked to oxidative stress and are co-factors for heart disease, which is why there are so many sugar-free diets now being implemented in mainstream medicine and health. Elevated insulin levels can lead to increased ovarian and adrenal androgens (male hormones) and triglycerides, and decreased HDL cholesterol (good cholesterol). An equilibrium cannot be maintained and so the cycle of PCOS symptoms continues.

Women with PCOS have an abnormal metabolism of androgens and oestrogen. PCOS can occur when there is an abnormal function of the hypothalamic-pituitary-ovarian (HPO) axis. If there are 12 or more follicles on one of your ovaries then you would be diagnosed with polycystic ovaries and not PCOS. Although the exact aetiology of PCOS is unclear, a primary characteristic is insulin resistance.

So let's just remind ourselves of what ovaries should look like. Women have two ovaries and the function of these is to produce eggs. Each month between 15 and 20 eggs mature inside the ovaries and the ripest egg is released and swept into one of the fallopian tubes. Women who have PCOS do not always ovulate, meaning that they do not always release egg cells – the follicles start to develop normally but they do not rupture and no eggs are released. As a consequence, multiple follicles and cysts are left in the ovaries. A cyst is just a large follicle that is roughly 25–30mm (1–1¼ inches) in diameter. The name polycystic ovaries simply means ovaries with many cysts.

What PCOS may look or feel like to you

Hirsutism: Don't be alarmed by the odd chin hair from time to time, it happens to us all. However, they grow when there is an increased level of male androgens, testosterone, so if you're getting lots of them it might be a sign of PCOS.

Acne/oily skin: These often go hand in hand when you have PCOS, as this condition raises testosterone levels and testosterone causes the sebaceous glands to produce too much of the oily sebum which gives you acne/spots.

Alopecia/baldness: Thinning hair due to the effects of male hormones (androgens) is called androgenic alopecia. It can be a major source of psychological distress to some women. This male-pattern hair loss is often seen in women with PCOS, congenital adrenal hyperplasia and other disorders that stem from male hormone excess. At the gut clinic I work with lots of women suffering from hair loss/thinning.

Weight gain: Weight is usually deposited on the abdomen, as this is where excess testosterone is laid down in men.

Amenorrhoea/oligomenorrhoea: Common in females who do a lot of endurance sport. Women with PCOS show menstrual irregularities that range from light to very heavy, irregular periods. The condition affects about 6 per cent of premenopausal women and is related to excess androgen production.

Sugar cravings: These are due to the influence of insulin, a powerful growth hormone and also an appetite stimulant, which can cause weight gain, and of course make it difficult to lose weight. PCOS is a vicious cycle for some women as you crave carbohydrates and on eating them this raises your blood sugar levels, which means more insulin is secreted, and too much insulin equals weight gain, making you insulin resistant. There's no question that sugar wreaks havoc on the health of women with PCOS. Not only does sugar spike insulin levels but it also contributes to high blood pressure, high levels of triglycerides and high levels of C-reactive protein, all of which has been linked to oxidative stress and inflammation.

So are women with PCOS powerless when it comes to sugar? Well, they can be unless they take action to control their sugar intake. Here's how to do it.

Other options for prevention of PCOS

Foods that contribute to PCOS	Foods to reverse and prevent PCOS
Processed sugars: All create drastic hormonal imbalances and the only way to reverse PCOS is to give up the processed sugars in fizzy drinks, processed foods and refined foods	**Complex carbohydrates:** Quinoa, sweet potatoes, brown rice, basmati rice and wild rice all help regulate blood sugar levels and slow the release of insulin
Alcohol: If you have any hormonal imbalances, alcohol is the first thing that you should give up. Alcohol loves oestrogen in the body and can cause hormone-receptor-positive breast cancer to grow and increase oestrogen levels. Just one drink a day doubles the risk of hormone-receptor-positive invasive breast cancer; the more alcohol a woman consumes, the more likely she is to develop this type of cancer[5]	**Iodine:** PCOS can also be caused by low iodine levels. You will get small amounts of iodine from fish but I recommend introducing nori seaweed, other sea vegetables or kelp flakes into your diet to optimise levels
Caffeine: This is another chemical that can impair sex hormones in the body and further add to the perpetual PCOS cycle. Be aware that some painkiller medications, fizzy and energy drinks can also contain high amounts of caffeine	**Fibre:** The great thing about fibre is that by consuming 35g (1¼ oz) or more a day you can dramatically reduce your chances (up to 70 per cent) of developing digestive-related cancers. Specifically for PCOS, fibre is important as it helps to bind and remove excess hormones from the body
Processed, fried and burnt meat: All meat that has preservative on and looks like Play-Doh, all burnt meat, all meat fried in oil. The exception is grass-fed, organic meat twice a week – eat this otherwise your body will not thank you	**Organic food:** The problem with pesticides is that they can have hormone-mimicking functions in the body. Not what you need when trying to reverse a hormone-related disease!

Other preventative measures for PCOS

Herbs, spices and supplements: Some herbs, spices and supplements will help regulate blood sugars and cravings, such as cinnamon, ginseng, berberine and chromium.

Exercise: If you are overweight, losing weight is essential, as it will improve your mood and overall health. Studies have shown that addressing weight loss can be very effective in regulating the hormonal imbalances associated with PCOS. Aim to do a 30-minute session three times a week – dancing, running, badminton, a gym class or hiking, it doesn't matter what, as long as you get your body sweating and your heart rate elevated.

Avoid stress: You must learn to develop anti-stress techniques. High stress levels can contribute to high insulin levels and other hormonal imbalances. Yoga is a great help here.

THE BEST FOODS FOR FERTILITY, FOR HIM AND FOR HER

Imbalanced blood sugar levels cause your hormones to be imbalanced; if you are wanting to conceive these are two foundational factors that need to be in balance and regulated, which is why they find themselves in this chapter on the pancreas.

If you are trying to get pregnant, think about how you and your partner can optimise your diets, sleep, supplement intakes, movement and lifestyle programmes. Creating a healthy environment is key to optimising your chances. Follow the recommendations here along with the rest of the guidelines for a healthy body – you should start seeing and feeling changes in three months or so.

Infertility is linked mainly to diet and lifestyle these days, unless there is a medical complication on one or other side of the partnership, so an overhaul of all the body's systems must be addressed. Taking care of your diet allows you to put yourself first and comes

THE BEST POSSIBLE YOU

with many other advantages, too. Many couples may experience sub-clinical (not severe enough to be a definite diagnosis) conditions which on their own will not be the root cause of infertility but all put together will contribute significantly to reducing the probability of conceiving. Take a lactose or gluten intolerance – neither will be the root cause but both may cause inflammation in the gut, which can minimise your nutrient absorption and lead to deficiencies. Nutrients are needed for healthy sperm, egg and hormone production, so optimal digestion is really the biggest factor in healthy hormones.

Then look at all the other exposures that the body is susceptible to, such as heavy metals and toxic chemicals on foods and drugs – all these can damage DNA. If we are in control of our gene expression and structure through diet and lifestyle, as research suggests, then we can be responsible for our own health.

Foods for him, foods for her

For him	Why	For her	Why
Oily fish	For the essential fatty acids that aid sperm development, enhancing quality and mobility	**Water**	For the reproductive system. If you're dehydrated, your cervical fluid (the stuff that helps the sperm find the egg) also becomes sluggish
Beans, nuts, seeds, eggs or oysters	For zinc levels 15mg a day minimum is essential for sperm repair	**Lean proteins**	Proteins are vital for egg production. Increasing protein intake is great for women in the lead-up to pregnancy, then once pregnant it can be decreased

Spinach	High in folate, improves sperm production	Orange fruits and vegetables	For vitamin A and beta carotene production, which helps produce the female sex hormones for ovulation
Avocado	For vitamin E, improving the quality of the sperm and full of unsaturated fats that are good for hormones	Nuts, seeds and oils	These are all extremely rich in essential fatty acids, which are crucial for healthy ovulation

Healthy sperm

For women, fertility may seem less complicated, because they are born with their egg quota, but for men sperm regeneration is approximately 75 days, so if you are living a chaotic life with many late nights, hours in front of the computer, and are relying on takeaways and alcohol, regeneration is not going to be optimal and will not be up to fertilisation. For fertilisation to happen, sperm need to be sprinting out of the blocks with vitality and gusto, which requires your body to be healthy and active.

Sperm disorders contribute to 40 per cent of infertility cases.

Miscarriages are not just down to the women, there are two people in this partnership. There are lots of things for the male to take a look at to help get to the root cause, such as getting a sperm test to check the amount and strength of the sperm, and again, it is important to make sure the diet and lifestyle choices of both partners is optimum.

If you have been told that the quality of your sperm or the quantity of your eggs is low and that's the way it is, you've been misinformed. It is possible to improve the quality of your eggs and sperm – it just takes

120 days for maturation. Everything that you and your partner eat or are exposed to will influence the health of the sperm and egg. A baby is a 50–50 product of his or her parents, who provide the genetic building blocks for the child from the moment of conception, as well as the generation and maturation of the gamete cells that form the embryo. Therefore, optimising the quality of eggs and sperm is of paramount importance, so it's crucial to follow a good preconception plan for a minimum of four months before trying to conceive. There are some care products that will adversely affect the quality of sperm, such as bisphenol A, which is used to coat foods, phthalates, which are most common in plastics, and organochlorine pesticides, which can most commonly be found on cereals and fruits. If you are having problems with fertility, being cautious of these products will most certainly help.

Of course, there will always be the chance that those pesky free radicals will get in the way and accumulate, but as long as you get enough antioxidants, vitamins and minerals from vegetables and fruits you will be in a better position to fight these off. Here are some guidelines:

- Always have something green on your plate at main meals.
- Drink 1.5 litres (2½ pints) of water every day.
- Do not eat any takeaways during the week.
- Take the supplements recommended on page 187.
- Twice a week, make a new recipe from scratch using ingredients that will increase your vitamin and mineral and microbiome diversity.
- Consider your beauty regime and the household products you buy to ensure you're not coming into contact with unwanted chemicals (see page 31).

How to increase fertility for him

Exercise
Strength training is the preferred gym exercise as it will boost

testosterone levels and reduce insulin resistance, which is what you want. If you have been told you have a low sperm count or are infertile you need to hit the weights, not pound the streets. Men who spend nine minutes a week lifting weights have a 25 per cent sperm count increase compared to those who do not. If you have weight to lose, do so if you want to conceive; research says that men who have a healthy weight have a higher sperm count than overweight men.

Nutrition

Increase your water intake: Water is essential for every metabolic function in the body. Eating excess sugar can often leave us thirsty, so avoid it and remember that feeling hungry is sometimes a sign of actually being thirsty.

Increase your intake of fruits and vegetables: Eat more of these foods because they are great sources of antioxidants that repair the damage of free radicals.

Decrease alcohol, drugs and smoking: None of these will contribute in a positive way to any health plan, so ideally they need to be eliminated. If this is one step too far, start by reducing your intake and perhaps work with a hypnotherapist or therapist to help you.

Supplements found in foods: The following will all help male fertility: zinc, which is best absorbed at night, is found in oysters and eggs and will help raise the male hormone testosterone; B12, which is again found in oysters and oily fish and is essential for cell division; and vitamin C, which is found in all your dark leafy vegetables and fruits and helps the sperm bind to the egg.

Lifestyle

Manage your stress: Not being able to get pregnant is another stress on the body, but worrying about it will only make matters worse. I say to couples that this is a great time to get your body into the healthiest place it can be and the bonus will be getting pregnant. This is your time to look after you, so put yourself first and enjoy the process.

Keep your balls cool: Sperm are finely tuned baby-making machines and they require a temperature that is 4°C (39°F) cooler than the rest of the body in order to make this happen. They achieve this by having a muscle called the cremaster muscle. When the temperature drops, the muscle contracts and pulls the testicles in close to the rest of the body. When the temperature gets warmer, the balls relax and hang. Sperm do not like warm temperatures. Sperm don't like it when you cross your legs, either!

How to prevent infertility for her

Exercise

Keeping active is important, but it is also important not to overdo it as this can leave you tired and stressed and can put more pressure on your adrenal glands and body fat percentage. Make sure you exercise sensibly, which means trying to decrease body fat at a time when you want to get pregnant will not help your fertility chances.

Nutrition

Eat the rainbow: Make sure you have good lean proteins and fats in your diet, along with leafy greens and brightly coloured vegetables and fruits, to get the full spectrum of vitamins and minerals.

Alcohol consumption: There have been several studies on the effects of alcohol on monkeys and rats in laboratories that prove multiple fertility issues arise from alcohol consumption. These include amenorrhoea (absent or delayed cycle), reduced ovarian weight, lowered hormone concentrations, inhibited ovulation and interference with sperm cell transportation through the fallopian tube.

Lifestyle

Keep cool!: It's easy to feel stressed when you want to get pregnant but stress can decrease chances of conceiving. So look after yourself and do what makes you feel relaxed: read a book, listen to music – the list is endless if you let your imagination go.

Case study

A brave starling

Lucy was a client who always reminded me of a little bird that had fallen out of a tree. She was fragile, emotional, scared and at this point unhappy. Having said all this, she did a grand job at distraction. She knew what made her happy and she was excellent at drawing her focus to this. We all get sad sometimes and fall into the basket of negative rubbish, but the strong-minded pull themselves out of it and move on.

Lucy walked into the clinic one day looking 10 years older than she was. Her posture gave her away more than anything but in front of me stood a 39-year-old fragile starling wanting to get pregnant and have a child. She was one of many women and men who come to me to make sure that their nutrition is optimal and that they are doing everything right for a healthy conception.

Lucy had had a succession of miscarriages – the first at six weeks, then lost a second baby at 8–10 weeks, but she didn't find out until they saw there was no heartbeat at the 12-week scan. She had taken Cyclogest during all her pregnancies – progesterone is the active ingredient in Cyclogest, which is a hormone that occurs naturally in the female body. It is essential for the reproductive system; after ovulation, if an egg is not fertilised, the level of progesterone in the blood falls before a menstrual period starts. Some women find that using progesterone for

12–14 days before their period starts can relieve the symptoms of premenstrual syndrome. Progesterone helps to support and maintain the pregnancy by causing the lining of the womb to thicken in preparation for a fertilised egg to implant. If the pregnancy is confirmed after 12 weeks, progesterone production continues to support the pregnancy.

For her fourth pregnancy, which was when I met Lucy, she was on the highest dose of this drug possible and she took it orally, religiously. The Cyclogest really helped as her progesterone levels were very low during the first three pregnancies. She took a multivitamin twice a day and Floradix magnesium liquid for the first six months as she was having leg cramps during this time, which the magnesium addresses.

I will never forget Lucy walking in one day halfway through the wellness plan programme. She was a completely different woman. With a sharp new haircut and an upright posture, confidence and energy just oozed out of her. It was such a transformation from the lady who had walked into the clinic three months earlier.

Lucy followed her metabolic typing diet throughout the pregnancy. She shopped organically and sourced her food from as many independent and local butchers and fishmongers as possible. She was very much in control. Having a child meant more to her than anyone I had met.

Her consultant said that in his opinion it was the aspirin and the Cyclogest that did the work of carrying her baby through. Lucy thinks it was more a case of eating more really good-quality food at regular intervals and in small amounts.

Today she has a beautiful little girl who is her pride and joy.

TOP 10 TIPS FOR A HEALTHY PANCREAS

1. **Reduce your sugar intake:** The pancreas secretes hormones and digestive juices to help you break down food. If you overload the pancreas with sugar you will wear out your insulin levels, potentially leading to diabetes. An easy way to do this is to keep a diet diary for a week and highlight all the high-sugar foods, like chocolate, grains, biscuits and granola, then decide to find an alternative or cut down on your intake.

2. **Increase your hydration:** Every organ needs hydration and the pancreas is no exception. If you are well hydrated your sugar cravings and intake will be low and you will be looking after the health of your pancreas. Always wake up in the morning to a glass of water, or at the very least a sip.

3. **Drink garlic broth:** Garlic broth is an essential healer for the gallbladder, liver and pancreas, which all work in tandem for optimal health of all the organs.

4. **Cut down your alcohol intake:** Alcohol is a poison to the pancreas, liver and the gallbladder, so if you think you are drinking too much, you probably are. There must be more days in the week when you do not drink alcohol than you do; if this is not the case you will come up against health issues.

5. **Snack on red grapes for a sugar kick:** The sweetest non-toxic, non-caloric or low-calorie antioxidant sweetener may be erythritol, found naturally in pears and red grapes, which won't stimulate your insulin response.

6. **Eat cherries in season:** Cherries are filled with antioxidants and phytochemicals that protect your heart. When eaten daily, they have been shown to reduce inflammation.

7. **Juice vegetables:** Juice vegetables for an intravenous shot straight to the body. These are also low in sugar, so if you do have diabetes or pancreatitis, drinking green vegetable juices even once a week will

THE BEST POSSIBLE YOU

improve your vitamin, nutrient and sugar intake.

8. **Eat good fats:** Try to get all the fats you need from foods such as avocados, nuts and seeds, and natural fats from meat and fish.

9. **Ramp up your vitamin B:** B3, which is also known as niacin, and B5 are both known for their fat and carbohydrate metabolism. You can get all your B vitamins from the meat and the vegetables you eat.

10. **Eat kiwis:** These are apparently the best foods for your pancreas and are full of flavour. They are great in smoothies as they naturally sweeten things up. Make sure you buy organic as conventional ones just don't taste of anything.

Footnotes

(1) 'Endocrine regulation of glucose metabolism', www.rose-hulman.edu/~brandt/Chem330/EndocrineNotes/Chapter_5_Glucose.pdf (accessed on 21/02/2016).

(2) Harcombe, Z. et al, 'Evidence from prospective cohort studies did not support the introduction of dietary fat guidelines in 1977 and 1983: a systematic review', *British Journal of Sports Medicine* (2016).

(3) Public Health England, Eatwell Guide, www.nhs.uk/Livewell/Goodfood/Documents/The-Eatwell-Guide-2016.pdf (accessed on 21/01/2016).

(4) Middleton, T., *Women Beware Women*, (London, 1957).

(5) Cancer Research UK, 'Alcohol and breast cancer – how big is the risk?', scienceblog.cancerresearchuk.org/2017/05/25/alcohol-and-breast-cancer-how-big-is-the-risk/ (accessed on 21/03/2016).

6. THE LUNGS

Sadness and Grief

WHAT DO THE LUNGS DO AND WHERE ARE THEY LOCATED?

We draw breath an average of 23,000 times a day and yet while it is a necessity, air is not a commodity we can package. Each of us relies on our own lungs to filter out the pollution we breathe in from the outside world. Therefore, while air is available in plentiful quantities, some of us struggle to breathe it more than others. Nevertheless, every cell of our bodies needs it and without it, we die.

Located superiorly to the diaphragm and deep within the pleural cavity is the amazing pump house that is your lungs. The lungs work tirelessly night and day, bringing you oxygen from the air and excreting the waste product, carbon dioxide, to stop you poisoning yourself.

You have two lungs, and these bilateral organs are efficiently protected by a rack of bones – the ribs – which ensure that these vital pumps do not receive any punctures.

The right lung has three lobes and the left lung has two, being slightly smaller because of the space taken up by the heart. Inside the lungs are your bronchi, which look like tree roots. At the end of each bronchus, known as a breathing tube, are your bronchioles and at the end of these are your alveoli, which are little sacs resembling flowers. The alveoli are extremely important as this is where the exchange of gases takes place. It is from these air sacs that oxygen is absorbed into the blood, while carbon dioxide, the waste product, is exhaled.

The lungs are covered by a layer of thin tissue called the pleura, the same type of tissue that surrounds the chest cavity. Between the chest lining and the pleura is a layer of fluid that acts as a lubricant, so the lungs are able to glide freely and expand with each individual inhalation.

Facts:

- The lungs are the only organs in the body that are composed almost entirely of air.
- The lungs make the human body float in water.
- A human sneeze can travel up to 16kph (10mph).
- The right lung in humans is larger than the left, which has to accommodate the heart.

A BIT MORE ANATOMY

The lungs are pyramid-shaped, a paired organ connected by way of the right and left bronchi to the trachea. At the base of the lungs is the diaphragm. The diaphragm assists breathing along with the intercostal muscles, which are small muscles that lie crisscrossed between the ribs. They are integral to the lung function. I once ended up in A&E from straining my intercostal muscles and diaphragm, one of the most painful things I have experienced; it didn't help that I was on a first date at the time – hyperventilating, pallor and shivering are generally not considered a good look.

The diaphragm makes up part of your 'core', along with the transverse abdominals, the erector spinae muscles and the pelvis. The core is not all about the strength of your rectus abdominis but the strength of your entire body, with the anal sphincter and your big toe being two of the most influential stabilisers. As the diaphragm contracts it increases the length and diameter of the chest cavity and expands the lungs. The nervous system plays a role here, too, as the muscles used in breathing can only contract when the nerves connecting them to the brain are intact. In injuries of the brain, such as a stroke, the nervous connections between the brain and the diaphragm are interrupted, leaving only the option of artificial ventilation to save the day.

The pleurae: The pleura layers allow the lungs to move with ease within the thoracic cavity. There are two pleurae: the visceral pleura is a slippery membrane which covers the surface of the lungs, dipping into the areas separating the different lobes of the lungs, while the parietal pleura lines the thoracic wall and the diaphragm. The facing surfaces of the parietal and visceral pleurae slide smoothly against each other during respiration, but when the pleura becomes inflamed it creates a condition called pleurisy.

The respiratory system: This has built-in methods to prevent harmful substances in the air entering the lungs. Hairs in your nose help filter out large particles – tiny little hairs called cilia (found along the air passages) move in a sweeping motion to keep the air passages clean. The cilia can get damaged (for example, from cigarette smoke) and stop functioning properly, which can lead to bronchitis. The mucus that one from time to time coughs up carries impurities out of the body. The mucus cells lining the bronchial tubes function to trap bacteria, viruses and allergy-causing substances and all other free radicals and reduce the chances of these harmful substances entering deep into the lungs. So, as gross as it may look and sound, the age-old adage is true – better out than in – spit out that mucus!

Did you know?

Aleix Segura Vendrell (Spain) currently holds the world (male) record for holding his breath with a time of 24 minutes and 2.45 seconds in 2016.

The average person can hold their breath for 30 seconds, so this is quite some record![1]

ENERGIES OF THE LUNGS

The meridian of the lungs

The lung meridian controls the breath and starts at the anterior aspect of the arm and forearm, ending near the thumbs (chest, inner arm and thumb tip), and it can affect your sense of smell, sinuses, mucus production and skin. If the lung meridian is out of balance you may experience a chronic cough, chest discomfort, breathing difficulty, sore throat, fever, flu, asthma and bronchitis.

Properties of the lung meridian

Force: Yin (female)

Chakra: Heart – love and relationships

Organ body clock: 3–5am

Season: Autumn

Colours: White and light blue

Fragrances: sweet and minty

Metaphysical lesson: Letting go

The energies of the lungs

Every breath you take is a gift of life; breathe in the new and breathe out the old. Take every day one step at a time. Build the life that you crave, that you want, that you deserve. Fear will create insecurity, then dreams will be hard to reach.

Having a strong pair of lungs is often something we say about a physically robust figure. It gives the impression of strength and vitality. A powerful voice is common with a strong pair of lung energies (or Qi) and both complement each other. This person is a picture of health with a strong immune system and an ability to recover from illness quicker and more effectively. A strong posture enables the lungs to be strong, and a welcoming chest encouraging communication will follow, inviting conversation and openness. This open posture reflects a strong sense of self-worth and respect, stepping forward with ease and confidence into the world.

If the energy of the lungs is weak, health imbalances in the immune system will start to show. Breathing dysfunction will be present and the person may display a forward head posture and open-mouth breathing; there may also be imbalances such as asthma and bronchial issues. A weaker immune system may result in longer healing times and also an inability to adapt to change. Personal boundaries may be weak, with a sadness and lack of confidence that seeps over into romantic and family relationships. People with weak lung energies find it hard to claim their plot of land in the world.

The emotions of the lungs

In traditional Chinese medicine the emotion most associated with the lungs is grief and sadness. Grief moves in like a sniper in a war zone. Often you have been fighting for so long that you know grief is inevitable but you are no more prepared for its arrival. At certain times in life we will experience loss in many ways; it is a rite of passage. Over time, we lose family members, friends and animals to death, but we also lose people in our lives when moving house, leaving school, university and jobs and because of differences in our needs and values. Grief is an emotion that it is important to feel but it is equally important to let go of; part of our journey through life is learning to appropriately let go of these emotions. Like snipping the branches of a tree for new flowers to blossom, this is true of new beginnings in life, too. Embrace the new beginnings rather than mourn the end of the old.

THE FOUR BODIES OF THE LUNGS

The spiritual body

The lungs are as light as spirit, with their thin membranes expanding to give breath and life to the rest of the body. Expanding into the alveoli like the flowers of purple sprouting broccoli, drawing in oxygen and leaking carbon dioxide, the lungs keep giving.

It is said that the lungs are archetypally related to the father figure. Lessons of self-value are associated with this organ, which help us as individuals to find our own place and value in the world. When we have been lucky enough to have these teachings it helps later in life with setting boundaries and having a separation from our mother. Good fathering teaches this boundary and helps us to understand who we are and what we are doing here on Earth. The lungs are associated with self-esteem and when this inner self-belief is lacking, fear becomes the emotion that starts to manifest into tissues of the body, creating disease states. When a boundary is strong, communication is strong and we can express ourselves outwardly; when the boundary is weak, chaos ensues. The ability to say what we mean, and to say yes when we mean yes and no when we mean no, is not only liberating but a very basic essential skill that we need in order to have clarity about who we are and what we want.

Action: Sit on the edge of your chair with your feet shoulder width apart. Put your hands on your thighs with your palms facing up. Lift both arms with palms facing upwards above your head and look up towards the sky. To make the lung sound, start by taking a deep breath, then with a slow exhalation make the 'sssssssssss' sound while exhaling almost 75 per cent of the air in your lungs. As you inhale, visualise energy entering into the lungs again and repeat. The sound should be gentle and calm.[2]

The emotional body

The lungs like to be clean and free of clutter and this is represented in the emotional body, too. The season of the lungs is autumn, a good time to clean up your environment and look at all the aspects of your life that need attending to. The lungs are nourished by respect; self-respect is a huge health supplement for these organs. Clearing up unfinished business can externally support the lungs and bring more clarity into your life, emotionally and mentally. A well-maintained and respected home and self are expressions of lung energy. The lungs are also associated with attachment, so people with weak lung energy may find it hard to let go of people or things and may spend an amount of time talking about the past. If the energy of the lungs is weak you may find yourself in a state of depression and the blues.

Action: Give your house, windows and drawers a good clean. Throw out everything that is cluttering your life and keep all the things that bring value to you. You will soon find that you have thrown out a lot of things you didn't think you needed. Put them on eBay or take them to a charity shop; your throwaway will always be another's gift.

The nutritional body

The key to healthy lungs is making sure they are unburdened by foods that the body finds hard to break down. Making sure your diet is clean, fresh and organic will minimise the strain on your breathing apparatus. Fresh, raw foods are the best way to get the enzymes, vitamins, minerals and antioxidants that will keep you breathing easily. Mucus-forming foods such as milk, cream and yoghurt were referred to by the ancient Greeks as the phlegmatic humour. In traditional Chinese medicine, dairy products are not recommended for the lungs for the same reason, because they cause congestion and build up phlegm.

Action: Make sure you drink water for its cleansing qualities. Pure clean water is essential for keeping the blood flowing to and from the lungs as well as helping them stay hydrated and keep the mucus flowing. Although we see mucus as something we don't want, it plays an important role in assisting toxins, microbes and pollutants to be expelled from the body. Maintaining a healthy diet supplemented with vitamins C and E, zinc and cod liver oil helps to prevent the build-up of mucus.

The physical body

The best way to improve the efficiency and the function of the lungs is to ensure they breathe in fresh unpolluted air and that you deepen the physical capacity of the lungs. The lungs rely on the diaphragm for function, but any improvement of the cardiovascular system makes it easier for the lungs to do their job.

Action: A few minutes each day of relaxed breathing, learning to breathe by engaging the diaphragm and relaxing the muscles of the chest and shoulders, can be a very effective way to increase the capacity of the lungs. Exercise the lungs every day to get the breath pumping and increase the efficiency of oxygen delivery around the body. Even by making some changes to your lifestyle you can improve the health of your lungs. Take the stairs instead of the escalator, walk instead of taking the car, walk to the next bus stop instead of getting on at your usual one. Take off your shoes and put your hands on your ribs; allow the breath to move your hands away from the centre of your body and as you breathe out allow your hands to come in and your tummy to pull tight to your back. Repeat 10 times.

Exercise nourishes the lungs like water nourishes a rose.

HOW TO KEEP YOUR LUNGS HAPPY

Your lungs will love you if you eat and drink foods that enable you to breathe freely, such as mint, peppermint and eucalyptus oils and green vegetables, and keep yourself hydrated with water, herbal teas, freshly squeezed fruits and cold-pressed juices. Your lungs like five-star hygiene environments. Time spent in the outdoors will get you bonus points with your lungs.

SIGNS THAT YOUR LUNGS ARE UNDER STRESS OR UNHAPPY

A cough that does not go away or gets worse: We all cough from time to time but a persistent cough should never be left untreated. This is because the lungs are warm and moist and can easily harbour infection. If you have been coughing for longer than a week and you do not have a cold or flu, it's advisable to seek medical attention.

Frequent chest infections: These infections usually occur because the body's immune system is compromised by its unrelenting fight against malignancy. If you suffer from chronic lung infections it is probably time for a chest x-ray.

Coughing up blood or rust-coloured sputum (spit or phlegm): Coughing up blood in phlegm is never healthy, even when it's just tiny spots of rust-coloured blood. In many cases coughing up blood is accompanied by other symptoms, including shortness of breath, a persistent fever or a pain in the chest. As a general rule of thumb, it's a good idea to make a doctor's appointment if you detect small amounts of blood in your phlegm, but seek immediate medical attention if you cough up a large volume of blood or if the bleeding doesn't stop.

Nutritional plan for a healthy pair of lungs

The food you eat impacts the health of your lungs, so choose wisely.

Meals and snacks	Nutrition	Benefits
On waking in the morning	Fresh mint and lemon in a teapot with filtered water	Refreshing, revitalising and regenerating
First meal of the day	**Grapefruit and pomegranate:** ½ grapefruit with sprinkled pomegranate seeds, pumpkin seeds and chia seeds	Full of vitamin C and antioxidants
Mid-morning snack, if desired	**Green juice:** Apple, kale, lemon and ginger	Detoxifying and easy on the digestive system
Second meal of the day	Cayenne pepper, red pepper and carrot soup with salmon flakes	Great inflammation busters
Mid-afternoon snack	5 x pineapple chunks and a chamomile tea	Calming and a sweet treat. Pineapple contains bromelain, a digestive enzyme, as well as vitamin C
Third meal of the day	A bowl of steamed onions, peppers, leafy greens, celery, parsley, garlic, horseradish, lemon, watercress, broccoli, tomatoes with grilled fish on the bone (trout, sea bass, snapper)	Full of detoxifying, antibacterial properties which help clear the airways

Bedtime snack / activity	Menthol steam bath: Put 3–4 drops of peppermint oil (see below) or tea tree oil in a hot bowl, put a cloth over your head and breathe	A decongestant to help clear sinuses and congested lungs

Peppermint for the lungs

The expectorant action of peppermint can help clear the lungs, so it is a useful herb to have in the garden or to have as an essential oil in the bathroom cupboard. The perennial peppermint plant has purple veins running through the leaves and tiny purple flowers in the summer months. As a medicinal herb, mint has been used for centuries for digestive complaints, although these days we see it mainly as a component of toothpastes.

When applied to the skin peppermint is refreshing and cooling, then gently warming. Its stimulating and analgesic properties make it an effective remedy for neuralgia, nausea and headaches.

PATHOLOGIES OF THE LUNGS

Pulmonary embolism: a blood clot on the lungs

A pulmonary embolism (PE) is a sudden blockage of the artery in the lungs, usually caused by a blood clot. It can be difficult to know when your body is about to fall out of balance in such a dramatic way, and there would be no way of pre-empting a PE. Sometimes as a result of a PE, the blood clots can cause scarring to the lungs, and at other times the clots can be deadly.

PE is not helped by being inactive or sitting for long periods of time at a desk, on long-haul flights or by being bedridden. These all increase the chances of clotting and deep vein thrombosis (DVT). You are also at higher risk for blood clots if you are an older adult (especially older than 70) or extremely overweight.

When clots form in the arteries they restrict the blood flow to the organs. When blood flow is restricted the high pressure in the arteries can eventually cause the clot to detach and form an embolus which can then travel and block the main artery to one of the organs such as the lungs, brain or heart with devastating consequences.

I experienced a PE at first hand with June. I knew her for 28 years, a time that was too short. I was probably seven when we met and 14 when our relationship started to blossom. If June was a tour de force, her husband Jim was the pièce de résistance, an academic, scientist and surrogate grandfather – I always seemed to do well in science projects at school thanks to Jim! Jim was always there on the sideline watching my sister and me play hockey when Dad was away, and the couple always reserved their Friday nights for gin and tonics and a good old natter/gossip at Pebbledash (their house), often with my family there. I later came to realise that gin and tonic on Fridays was actually therapy, disguised. Jim and June were family, friends, and, in fact, meant more to me than words can express. They were there for all the major moments in my life and their home was invariably the first stop I would make on my visits back to Somerset. So when the phone call came early one Friday evening in February 2014, a sense that something was not right swept over me. All I needed to hear was the tone of my mum's voice to know that she was about to deliver some bad news. June had died of a pulmonary embolism. Sudden, no build-up, tragic.

The worst thing about these types of death is that someone is taken from you in an instant. She had had a cold, but the first sign that she was really under the weather was that she was off her whisky. It's funny how we learn the traits of our nearest and dearest and how they can be greater markers in health than a blood test. We joked about it – that she must be ill if the evening Glenfiddich was being given the night off. On the last trip to the quiz night at the local village pub, which was a stone's throw away, Jim drove. Both of them were fit and active residents of the village and it would have taken longer to get the car out than to walk, so this was another sign that all was not well. And then, with no further sign, she fell and was gone.

What a blood clot might look or feel like to you

Vital signs of life, such as heart rate, breathing rate and blood pressure, can all be normal if you have PE, but depending on the size of the blood clot or just how much lung tissue has been affected the vital signs can also be abnormal. Abnormal vital signs are actually classic signs of PE.

If there is a blood clot on the lungs you may experience the following symptoms:

- An elevated heart rate (tachycardia).
- A cough that produces blood (haemoptysis).
- Elevated respiratory rate (tachypnoea).
- Fast, rapid breathing.
- Discolouration (bluish tinge) of the skin and mucous membranes (cyanosis) due to decreased oxygen saturation, which is basically when red blood cells do not have oxygen attached to them.
- Decreased blood pressure (hypotension).

Red flags that require immediate medical attention:

- A wash of anxiety or a sensation of lightheadedness which can come with shortness of breath.
- Severe chest pain that becomes worse on every breath you take.
- Coughing up blood.

The heart rate and the respiratory rate both elevate as the body tries to compensate for less oxygen transfer in the lungs and work harder to distribute oxygen to the body's organs and tissues. This can in turn lead to a lightheadedness and a weakness as the body's organs are being deprived of the oxygen they need to function. In some cases the blood clot can block blood from the right side of the heart, preventing blood getting to the lungs which can result in shock (circulatory col-lapse) and sudden death.

In 25 per cent of PE cases clients experience sudden death – they collapse, their breathing halts and their heart stops beating, which is known as cardiac arrest, and all without prior symptoms. PE is the second leading cause of sudden death after coronary heart disease.

Other ways to help prevent pulmonary embolism

Assess your life: Have you got your life in order so that you can successfully let go of the things/people in it that no longer bring you light? If this is not the case, start by addressing your boundaries. Daily meditation can help bring focus and order into your life. Start slow and small and build up. Sit in a quiet place, in a comfortable position, and focus on something in your life that is positive and that you feel confident about. Close your eyes and allow this thought to absorb this moment for 2 minutes. The moment another thought pops into your head, take a deep breath and start again or allow that to have been your meditation for the day. Over the coming days and weeks build this time up so that you can focus on the positive in your life without your mind jumping around.

Move: Do not let your body get stagnant; move every day. Walking is the best exercise for the lungs as you can regulate how much you want to work them. The fresh air in the lungs brings up debris and mucus that are not welcome and the cardiovascular system gets a workout, too. Find a time in your day to allocate 10 minutes to get moving and work up from there to get your lungs pumping, your breath puffing, your skin sweating and your muscles moving – your body will feel fantastic for it. If you spend a lot of your time inside, try to get outside to do this exercise.

Diet: The nutritional plan for healthy lungs on page 202 is a perfect diet to follow. There are also some supplements you can take. Ginkgo biloba has been found to help by reducing fibrin content, which is a protein involved in forming blood clots; and bromelain fights blood clotting by stopping the platelets sticking together on the walls of the blood vessels; both vital factors in preventing heart attacks and strokes. Bromelain is a protease enzyme found in the stems of pineapples, which is why you often get a pineapple with your gammon steak, as the bromelain helps break down the protein. Try adding fresh pineapple to your meat dish or take a bromelain supplement; it should also improve your digestion.

Asthma

If you read about asthma online you will come across a lot of information that says the cause is unknown. While this is true, what happens physiologically if you have asthma is known. So let's look at the physiology before the pathophysiology to get a better picture of just exactly what asthma is, apart from being a problem with breathing! You will be pleased to learn that it is more preventable than you might have been led to believe.

Asthma is a chronic inflammatory disease of the airways. As with every individual and every pathology, the signs and symptoms differ. What is consistent with this condition is that when the airways come into contact with a trigger they become inflamed and react by narrowing, so it is essential that the bronchi secrete mucus to trap the bacteria and other foreign materials that may get into the alveoli. Mucus is an inflammatory response; just like when you are ill with a cold or the flu, it is a vehicle to clear unwanted substances out of the body.

When this happens, to a large degree, this is what's known as an asthma attack. The entrance to the airway, and therefore breathing, is now restricted and creates that common shortness of breath (SOB), coughing to clear the mucus and wheezing. The cough is the body's attempt to clear the mucus inside the airway, but unless you cough it up you either just dislodge it or swallow it into the stomach.

How to prevent asthma

1. **Have a food intolerance test.** There are some foods that cause an immediate reaction in the body; these are usually the main allergens, including gluten, eggs, soy, nuts and wheat. The reason these foods are the main culprits for digestive complaints and breathing difficulties is because they are the most widely eaten, especially in the Western diet. The majority of Westerners are brought up on a combination of these foods, which deplete the specific enzymes responsible for breaking down the proteins in them.

2. **Reduce dairy foods:** Dairy foods create the most noticeable effect on breathing for some people, because in the absence of the lactase enzyme which is present in so many of us, the protein is not broken down and remains as a strong allergen. Dairy foods that create the most noticeable mucus response are milk, cheese, yoghurt, ice cream, milk chocolate and all milk chocolate products.

3. **Optimise your vitamin D levels.** Low vitamin D levels correlate with asthma, and this deficiency is also at the core of many disease and ill-health states. The good news is that this couldn't be easier to rectify; all you have to do is get these tested with a health practitioner or your doctor, who, if your levels are low, will then prescribe you vitamin D3. Optimal vitamin D levels are also markers of good lung health, which is another good reason to take vitamin D. It is recommended by Public Health England that you take 10mcg of vitamin D every day in winter or if you are house- or office-bound and do not have a lot of sun exposure.[3]

4. **Reduce your omega 6 intake.** We all know about omega 3, they are the fish oils that reduce inflammation, but remember that omega 6 is not as friendly. These oils increase inflammation and can contribute to asthma, and it is the ratio between the two that is the problem. You will find omega 6s in processed and takeaway foods.

5. **Drink raw milk.** The difference between raw milk and regular milk is the pasteurisation process, and studies show that drinking raw milk not only helps reduce the incidence of asthma but also cuts down digestive problems and mucus production. The Parsifal Study, published

in 2007, and using data taken from 15,000 children, also found the consumption of raw milk was inversely associated with asthma and 'may offer protection against asthma and allergy'[4].

6. **Breastfeed your children if you can.** Breastfeeding has been shown to help protect against respiratory infections in early life.[5]

Other ways to help prevent asthma

Don't push yourself too much: When an individual has a chronic disease state such as asthma, the condition may prevent them taking part in activities they used to do, or they do so to a lesser extent, so take this into consideration.

Exercise your lungs: Find some breath-building exercises that expand the strength and capacity of the lungs. Put your hands gently around your ribs and allow the breath to expand your hands. Do this with a partner or a friend and see how much capacity the lungs actually have. If you see the shoulders rise or the face frown, relax and start again so that there is only movement visible in the ribs.

Salt-inhaling: One of my favourite things to do for easy breathing is to try some salt air therapy. There is no arguing that we all feel better after a day at the beach and a swim in the ocean, and these salt-filled, salt-lined rooms reflect this, acting as a powerful aid for people affected by breathing-related conditions. The ancient Ayurvedic and yogic cultures of India relied on salt-inhaling therapies to cleanse the nose and throat areas. The benefits of salt inhalers are vast, but here are just a few:

- May help lower blood pressure.
- Deepens breath capacity.
- Detoxifies the air.
- Boosts lung capacity and respiratory health.
- Reduces swelling and redness in the body.

Try supplements: There are several supplements which can help, too:

Magnesium is important in supporting the physical body; it helps promote the parasympathetic activity in the body and relaxation, which can help improve lung function and also relieve an acute asthma attack. Too much ingested magnesium will cause the digestive system to have too strong a parasympathetic drive, though, leading to diarrhoea, so adjust the dose accordingly. It is recommended you take 200–400mg in divided dosages three times a day, depending on your needs, so always check with your health practitioner.[6]

NAC (N-acetylcysteine) helps decrease the severity and frequency of asthma attacks by increasing glutathione (amino acid) and thinning bronchial mucus.

Quercetin is a natural antihistamine and anti-allergenic, like those found in citrus fruits, which has been shown to reduce the severity of exercise-induced asthma.

Levels of vitamin B6 can be low in people with asthma, but you can boost these by eating B6-rich foods such as wild-caught tuna, lean proteins, hazelnuts and cooked spinach. Its benefits in cardiovascular health are important, as vitamin B6 helps convert a compound called homocysteine into the amino acid cysteine. High levels of homocysteine in the blood have been connected to an increased risk of heart attacks and stroke.

The giant roundworm (*Ascaris lumbricoides*)

Ascaris lumbricoides is found in humans all over the world but more commonly in tropical and sub-tropical regions. It is estimated that 200 million people are infected with this roundworm, which is 2.5 per cent of the world's population. *Ascaris* likes to hang out in the lungs, but also the liver, heart, small intestines, pancreas, oesophagus and mouth and gains entry via the mouth or the nose.

The giant roundworm, which can grow to 15–45 centimetres (6–18 inches) in length – with the female being longer than the male – is the most common nematode known to humans and likes to hide out in the lungs, among other places. You can become infected with *Ascaris* by simply swallowing food that is infected – some of the larvae fall off the eggs, you then ingest them and become infected. If you do not have great HCL acid levels the larvae will get through the acid pool of the stomach and into the small intestine, then they will burrow out of the small intestines into the circulatory system, gaining access to the whole of the body. The larvae will then usually head towards the heart and into the lungs where they will grow into tiny worms, and every four or so weeks you will get a dry cough. This cough comes about when the worms have had enough of being in the lungs and decide to go back into the small intestines. When you cough you bring up the infection, then you swallow the worms back into the small intestines, where they can grow to 45 centimetres (18 inches) long and multiply to up to as many as 20 in a nest at a time. Parasites are very sociable and like to hang out in large groups together, and if they are present in those numbers they can cause blockages.

Most people who have an infection of *Ascaris* have few digestive symptoms but have a cough that just won't go away. Often a cough is dismissed as not being a symptom of anything at all, maybe of just being a little under the weather. If the infection is moderate to heavy the infestation – depending on the body part – will carry different symptoms and therefore will be slightly easier to diagnose.

Parasites are not uncommon and ultimately they have one goal, which is to reach the brain. When they have done this, if they haven't already, they will affect your emotions and in some cases can be mistaken for a brain tumour. Their plan is to manipulate the host in a way that will ensure their survival so they can reproduce, and as many parasites can outsmart antibiotics, especially if they have been living inside you for some time, finding a natural way to kill parasites is essential for mental health.

What the giant roundworm might look or feel like to you

Often the infection can live symbiotically with you as the symptoms are very mild, which can be the case with parasites, fungi and pathogenic bacteria.

Abdominal pain: Large infestations of worms can cause abdominal pain and intestinal obstruction. During the lung phase of larval migration, pulmonary symptoms can occur such as coughing, heartburn (dyspepsia), coughing up of blood (haemoptysis) and increased number of eosinophils (blood cells) in the blood (pneumonitis).

Oedema: An abnormal accumulation of fluid can build up in the lower body, specifically the hips.

Allergic reactions: When the parasite releases toxins into the bloodstream people can complain of eye pain, skin rashes and insomnia.

Reduced absorption: The three macronutrients – fat, protein and carbohydrate – are often inhibited with an *Ascaris* infection, as well as vitamin A.

Lactose intolerance: A symptom of *Ascaris*.

Cough: A persistent cough that can't be cleared.

Things that help if you have giant roundworm

Clear negative emotions: Parasites are masters of disguise and can mimic many vibrations of organ systems in the body. They thrive in environments that are stagnant, where there is congestion in the body and negative thoughts and patterns. When you do have an infection, take efforts to understand where these negative emotions come from in order to clear them. Write down on a piece of paper the first three negative emotions that plague your mind, then write next to them some suggestions for how you can make a change in the right direction.

For example:

Insecure thought: I'm not smart enough.

Owned thought: I am smart; this feeling of insecurity means that I want to further my learning and my journey or life, as I am inquisitive and curious. As I seek new information and experiences I allow myself to take a rest and be clear about my next step.

Supplements: As a rule of thumb, the following supplements all support a healthy body, but make sure you include one plant-based organic supplement, too. I like the range by Innate.[7]

- Multivitamin that contains copper
- Immune support
- Antioxidants
- B6
- Liver support
- Probiotics

Case study

It started with a sneeze

Every time a certain wine grape was drunk, endless sneezing followed. This went on for a number of years, much to the annoyance of the sufferer's family, and any empathy soon vanished as the cacophony of sneezing lost its charm and became irritating. The family's response after the tenth sneeze would be, stop drinking Chardonnay!

An immune response to the grape or the sulphites in the wine perhaps? A home intolerance test was taken by removing the wine and, sure enough, the sneezing came to a stop. The family gave a sigh of relief!

Coughs can be dry, chesty, tickly or sore. We all cough – some more than others – and we all clear our throats every day of our life. However, my experience of a cough becoming far more than just a little irritating was personal – it was my mother who was coughing.

While any cough that cannot be cleared is annoying – to the sufferer and those around them – this one took her to the verge of choking, leaving her gasping for breath. It continued on and off for two years. Then at 5am one morning, coincidentally, the day before an appointment with the doctor, she had what can only be described as a seizure of the brain. Locked jaw, dribbling mouth, stiffness, murmuring and then 20 minutes later back to reality.

The doctor immediately said it was an epileptic fit, although at 64 she had no previous history. She was taken off the road for six months as a precaution (a standard procedure). Lung x-rays were taken which confirmed an infection and a collapsed lung, and amoxicillin was prescribed. The MRIs came back clear, as in due course did the second x-ray on the lung, but she was still coughing. She was given no reason for the collapsed lung or explanation for what the infection was.

I recommended testing for bacteria, fungi and parasites in the GIT as I felt the cause of both the cough and the seizure hadn't been established. All disease begins in the gut – Hippocrates said this, not me, and quite some time ago! With a fully functional gut you are always closer to full health, so a persistent cough is a red flag and now, with a clear lung x-ray, I knew we had to look elsewhere. But, as happens in life, some things take precedence and there was devastating news when my aunt, my mother's sister, was diagnosed with motor neurone disease, so, for my mother, her sister's needs became paramount. This was obviously a dreadful period, with my aunt's condition rapidly deteriorating and my mother by her side at every step of her journey. Naturally, under such circumstances, lack of sleep, appetite and peace of mind are par for the course for both patient and carers.

And then, just one week away from the six-month mark, when Mum would have been allowed to resume driving, and while I happened to be staying with them, Mum had another seizure at 5am. A truly alarming thing to see! We headed for A&E. Four weeks later, it happened again. But one thing was oddly clear, the seizures invariably happened at the same time of day.

The lung is responsible for moving the Qi (energy) through the meridians and around the entire body, as well as providing immune protection. It is known that the lungs repair themselves and are most active between the hours of 3 and 5am. It is also a fact that there is a correlation between the lungs and the emotions associated with grief. It is why people report waking at these times when they are struggling with sorrow or loss. Physical manifestations of stress and imbalance may also show up as wheezing, coughing, asthma or getting sick easily.

My suggestion to my mother was that she start to do some emotional therapy to help her let go of the grief and trauma she was holding on to – her body was telling her something and she needed to listen. Talking to family and friends is helpful, but talking to a third party, who is trained to listen and hear, can be more healing. I suggested to her that tai-chi and acupuncture might also help to shift damaging energy from the body.

I was, however, convinced that the original diagnosis of adult onset epilepsy was incorrect, which was later borne out by a consultation with a neurologist. In summary, medical tests had shown my mother was healthy, but the continuing cough and seizures insisted something wasn't right.

It was at this point I came across a research paper – 'Blackout and Collapse in the Acute Setting', by Nicola Cooper.[8] A blackout or a collapse is how a client might describe what happened, but medically the diagnosis is 'Transient loss of consciousness' (TLOC). This paper discusses how many clients are admitted to hospital unnecessarily and not evaluated by following the evidence that has been presented. The initial evaluation is extremely important in diagnosing the cause of the collapse and should include an eyewitness account if possible. This paper focuses on initial evaluation and immediate management, then which tests should be ordered and which referrals made when no obvious diagnosis is immediately found.

Emotions cannot be ruled out as the seeds from which physical manifestations grow. Mental health and gut health create strong, robust physical health.

TOP 10 TIPS FOR HEALTHY LUNGS

1. **Learn how to breathe:** We all breathe – some more efficiently than others – and when you have mastered the art of breathing you will find that your organs thank you for it. When you breathe properly, your diaphragm, stomach and ribcage should expand harmoniously. Every cell in our body requires oxygen to survive. Proper breathing increases stamina, promotes mental clarity and better moods and helps the body detoxify more efficiently.

2. **Push your heart rate:** The more you work at your cardiovascular fitness, the more efficient your lungs will be at supplying your muscles and heart with oxygen. Push your body a bit further than usual and see how good it makes you feel.

3. **Release your diaphragm:** It's a wonderful holder of emotions and if

you are lucky enough and brave enough to have your diaphragm released, not only will you breathe with more ease, you'll feel lighter and emotionally more stable, too. Someone who practises NMT (neuromuscular therapy) or VM (visceral manipulation) will be able to do this technique. (Practitioner recommendations are at the back of this book.)

4. **Eat, juice and spice with cayenne pepper:** One of the many benefits or reasons to have more cayenne pepper in your life is its high capsaicin and beta carotene content. Cayenne pepper is an excellent decongestant and expectorant, which makes it useful in cystic fibrosis, where the transport of mucus is altered. It loosens phlegm or mucus from the lungs and airways, reduces swelling and inflammation on the respiratory tract, easing breathing problems and shortness of breath.

5. **Peel pistachios:** Pistachios are a good source of gamma-tocopherol. Eating them increases intake of gamma-tocopherol, so pistachios may help to decrease lung cancer risk.[9]

6. **Sign a clean air petition:** The world is simply getting more and more polluted, so do what you can on an individual level, because every little-bit does count. Drive less, Uber less, smoke less, use less electricity, burn less wood, light fewer fires. Whatever it is you do that produces pollution, endeavour to do it less. Do your bit!

7. **Take oregano oil:** A bottle of this oil should be in everyone's first-aid cupboard. It is a superhero for the respiratory tract and is now better at fighting the bacteria *Staphylococcus aureus* than common antibiotics. Its two compounds, carvacrol and rosmarinic acid, are both natural decongestants and histamine reducers that have direct, positive benefits on the respiratory tract and nasal passage airflow.

8. **Avoid pollution:** Your lungs are pretty durable if not attacked from the outside, and with COPD (chronic obstructive pulmonary disease) now one of the top causes of death in the world, we need to be aware of how much pollution we are actually breathing in. Get out to the country once in a while and breathe in the clean country air. It will do wonders for your whole body.

9. **Let go:** This is one of the best things you can do for the health of your lungs – emotionally, physically, mentally and spiritually. Acceptance of where you are is the only way to move on in life. Ask yourself what you want, then make a plan to go and get it.

10. **Eat your greens:** It has been proven that eating cruciferous vegetables can in fact lower the risk of lung cancer – but supplements do not count! Green foods keep your body alkaline, which is what we want. Disease does not like alkaline bodies to eat green and stay green.

Footnotes

(1) Longest time breath held voluntarily (male), www.guinness worldrecords.com/world-records/longest-time-breath-held-vol-untarily-(male) (accessed on 21/03/2016).

(2) Mantak, C., *Taoist Ways to Transform Stress into Vitality. The Inner Smile, Six Healing Sounds* (Huntington, NY, 1986).

(3) https://www.nhs.uk/conditions/vitamins-and-minerals/vitamin-d/#how-much-vitamin-d-do-i-need

(4) Food Safety News, 'Raw milk advocates stage "milk and cookies" protest at FDA', www.foodsafetynews.com/2011/11/raw-milk-advocates-stage-milk-and-cookies-protest-at-fda/#.WoxbIhP-FK8U (accessed on 21/01/2016).

(5) Bachrach, V.R.G., 'Breastfeeding and the Risk of Hospitalization for Respiratory Disease in Infancy', *Archives of Pediatrics & Adolescent Medicine* (2003).

(6) Pizzorno, J.E., *The Textbook of Natural Medicine* 4th Edn (London, 2012).

(7) Innate Response Formulas, www.innateresponse.com/ (accessed on 21/0/2017).

(8) Cooper, N., 'Blackout and Collapse in the Acute Setting', *Acute Medicine II* (London, 2016).

(9) American Association for Cancer Research, 'Pistachios may reduce lung cancer risk', www.sciencedaily.com/releases/2009/12/091208191956.htm (accessed on 23/01/2016).

7. THE HEART

Joy

As someone who is not trained or practised in listening to the beats and murmurs of the heart, my experience with this organ comes with emotional wounds, trials and tribulations. Of course, high blood pressure, elevated cholesterol and obesity all put pressure on the heart, which cause it to have to work harder, but there is an emotional side to the heart that will be my focus.

Wounds to the heart come in many packages, shapes and sizes and every client I see coming for weight-loss or digestive issues holds these wounds in a cradle of cotton wool. They are the most vulnerable clients that I see and even though they may be larger than life in their sunshine-like natures and personality, you just have to scratch a bit deeper and the wounds start to weep.

The heart is one of the most protected organs in the body, found deep in the pleural cavity, surrounded by the ribs. It is housed in the thoracic cavity, sitting slightly on the left and towards the midclavicular line, lying medially to the lungs and posterior to the sternum and surrounded by and protected by the ribs. Two-thirds of the heart's mass is found on the left-hand side, which is why it points to the left. The apex of the heart is in the fifth intercostal space, the space between your ribs.

Working away like a workhorse, never being allowed its beauty sleep until the last breath of air is pulled in, this fist-sized organ pumps not only life but love around your body in the form of blood, red blood cells and oxygen, which is all often taken for granted. It is the most talked-about and analysed organ and perhaps the only organ that is commonly associated with the emotional body, too.

Facts:

- The blue whale has the largest heart of all mammals, weighing 630kg (1,389 lb).
- The heart needs its own special blood supply from the coronary arteries.
- The heart has its own electrical impulse and so can beat outside of the body, providing it has an oxygen supply.
- In a lifetime, the heart muscle engages in more physical exercise than any other muscle.
- The heart starts to beat in a human embryo four weeks after conception.
- The heart pumps 7,500 litres (13,198 pints) of blood and beats over 100,000 times a day. In fact, the heart pumps 100,000 million gallons of blood through 96,560 kilometres (60,000 miles) of blood vessels in the human body – that's a lot of distance and liquid.

A BIT MORE ANATOMY

The heart functions as the body's circulatory pump, taking in de-oxygenated blood through the veins and delivering it to the lungs for oxygenation before it gets pumped back into the arteries.

The heart is encased in a wall that has three layers: the epicardium, myocardium and the endocardium. The epicardium is a thin layer of serous membrane that helps to lubricate and protect the outside of the heart. The myocardium makes up the majority of the mass of the heart, being the thickest layer, and is responsible for pumping blood.

The endocardium lines the inside of the heart and is responsible for preventing blood sticking to the inside of the heart and forming potentially deadly blood clots.

Inside the four chambers of the heart are a left and right atrium and a left and right ventricle. The right atrium pumps deoxygenated blood from the body to the right ventricle, which pumps the blood to the lungs to be oxygenated. The left atrium then pumps the oxygenated blood from the lungs to the left ventricle, which then pumps the blood around the body, about 5 per cent of which goes directly to the coronary arteries that supply the heart. The heart also has a connection system, which sets its own rhythm and signals to the rest of the body.

The route of the blood through the body to the heart and lungs may well be one you remember from school, but here is a simplified explanation: deoxygenated blood returns to the heart after travelling around the body, entering the superior and inferior vena cava. The blood enters the right atrium and is pumped through the tricuspid valve into the right ventricle. From here the blood is pumped through the pulmonary semilunar valve into the pulmonary trunk – it is the pulmonary trunk that carries the blood to the lungs where it releases carbon dioxide (which we don't want) and takes in oxygen (which we do want).

The blood in the lungs returns to the heart through the pulmonary veins and from here the blood enters the heart again via the left atrium. The left atrium contracts to pump blood through the bicuspid (mitral) valve into the left ventricle. The left ventricle pumps blood through the aortic semilunar valve into the aorta. From the aorta, blood enters into systemic circulation throughout the body tissues until it returns to the heart via the vena cava and the cycle repeats.

Did you know?

William Harvey was a physician who made seminal contributions to anatomy and physiology in the seventeenth century. He was the first to be able to describe systemic blood circulation and how blood was pumped to the brain and body by the heart. Before Harvey came Hippocrates, who greatly influenced Galen (a Greek physician, AD 130–210) with his theories and particularly 'the four humours', and posited that an excess or deficiency of any of the four distinct bodily fluids in a person directly influenced their temperament and health. The four humours are blood (air), yellow bile (fire), black bile (earth) and phlegm (water).

ENERGIES OF THE HEART

The meridian of the heart

The meridian of the heart starts at the axilla (armpit) and descends down the middle border of the arm, ending at the little finger of the hand. The heart meridian can affect the heart, speech, shoulder, circulation, perspiration and the tongue. If the heart meridian is out of balance you can experience chest pain, palpitations, angina, jaundice, pain in the arm, cardiac disorders, insomnia and hysteria.

Properties of the heart meridian

Force: Yin (female)

Chakra: Heart – love and relationships

Organ body clock: 11am–1pm

Season: Summer

Colours: Red, pink and gold

Fragrances: Rose and bitter aromas

Metaphysical lesson: Inner joy

The emotions of the heart

Today's modern society bombards us with electrical shocks of seven specific emotions more than ever before: anger, fear, fright, grief, joy, worry and pensiveness. Like the British weather, where four seasons appear in one day, so too can all these emotions.

The heart reacts in the same way to the tragic news of a loved one as it does in elation at a celebration: both cause shock. The heart is the emotional centre of the body; we say things like 'pour your heart out', 'I have a heavy heart', 'follow your heart', 'don't lose heart'.

If you look at the number of times each day we are exposed to shock/excitement in this society you can see just how easy it is for the heart to be in overdrive. The heart is overstimulated constantly – by the news, by social media, by human behaviour, by our obsession with being liked – all of these are stressful to the physiology of the body. TV shows, media, social media and magazines cause us to go from excitement to depression in minutes, forcing your heart to go on an emotional merry-go-round ride of feelings.

The heart actually just wants peace and tranquillity, as it is a busy little organ most of the day. If the heart is challenged by highs and lows all day long, diseased states of insomnia, depression, high and low moods and mania will all follow before too long.

THE FOUR BODIES OF THE HEART

The spiritual body

The energies of the heart are unique because the heart generates its own patterns of electrical fields, magnetic fields and electromagnetic energy. The heart and blood have the ability to affect the mental state of a person and their emotions.

Consciousness, sleep, memory and thinking are all affected by the state of the heart. If the heart is strong and the flow of blood and fluids is regular, normal mental activity and a balanced emotional life follows. If the heart is weak, the blood can be deficient and emotional highs and lows will be more common – such as depression, insomnia and a fog over life. When your heart is open you are a joy to be around as a person; you find it easy to receive love and equally to give love, and this is at the centre of the heart chakra.

Action: Try out sound healing for the heart. Qi (energy) is much more powerful and flowing in a body that is happy and laughs. Laughing is a fire sound and the heart is a fire organ, so laughing is the best medicine.

The emotional body

At the end of the day, the best information comes from the heart. If you are feeling in balance you will also be open-minded, peaceful and trustful of yourself and of others. When the exact opposite is true you may feel confused, doubtful and out of flow.

Action: Buy a colouring book or borrow your kids'! Find a quiet spot and colour for 20 minutes. You will find it hard to think about anything else while you are doing this, and this is what you need to do sometimes to find clarity of mind. Sometimes joy is to be found in the simplest of places – like a colouring book, which takes you back to childhood.

The nutritional body

The heart needs food that makes the blood flow easily around the body. It also needs foods that make you happy and can be easily digested. To prevent anything going wrong with the heart it is essential that it stays fit, and one of the best ways you can do this is by controlling your portion size. If you overload your plate with food, taking seconds to eat it and finishing feeling stuffed, you are overloading your body and your organs, and your heart has to do more work.

Action: Watch your portion intake, especially at restaurants, and eat smaller and lighter food in the evening – both of these things will help your heart and your waistline.

The physical body

Qi gong is primarily a discipline that focuses on integrating the breath with physical movement to create energy and flow. It is an ancient Chinese practice that has many health benefits, especially calming the mind and taking time for yourself.

Action: If you are experiencing palpitations, arrhythmias, high blood pressure and insomnia or sleep disturbances, there are some qi gong heart exercises that can help improve your heart's balance and circulation. With all qi gong exercises you will need to place your emphasis on the connection of your mind, breath and imagination.

Buddha's breath: As you inhale, extend your abdomen and fill it with air. As you exhale, contract your abdomen and expel the air from the bottom of your lungs. Inhale for a count of 10 and exhale for a count of 15. Do this 10 times. As you breathe in and out, imagine inviting your Qi energy to flow through your body.

HOW TO KEEP YOUR HEART HAPPY

Your heart loves it when you love unconditionally. It is equally important to look after our emotional health as our nutritional health. Be thankful for the life that you have and for the food that you have access to. When everything we do comes from a place of love there is no room for fear or anxiety.

Nutritional plan for a healthy heart

The key to a healthy heart is variety!

Meals and snacks	Nutrition	Benefits
On waking in the morning	Hawthorn berry tea	Refreshing, revitalising and regenerating
First meal of the day	Oats with almond milk, chia seeds and blueberries	Satisfying and full of good fats
Snack, if desired	Green tea leaves with freshly squeezed lemon	Lowers hypertension and is full of antioxidants[1]
Second meal of the day	Wild salmon, raw broccoli, pine nut and red onion salad with garlic and chilli flakes	High in omega 3s. Garlic is good for arterial health
Snack	Walnuts, raspberries with dark chocolate crumbles (broken-up 80% dark chocolate)	Full of heart-healthy polyphenols. Walnuts are high in omega 3s; magnesium, which is an essential mineral for the heart, is found in chocolate
Third meal of the day	Sardines (fresh) on dark rye toast with cherry tomatoes, rocket leaves and mustard greens	Sardines are loaded with omega 3s. Rye is full of magnesium, zinc and iron
Bedtime snack / activity	Magnesium salt bath with lavender and a square of dark chocolate	An oasis of happiness and love! All reducing anxiety and stress

The easiest thing to do with your diet when you are looking after the health of your heart in particular is to include fruits and vegetables that are native to the country you live in, eat lean proteins – mainly ones with a tail or two legs – and drink 2 litres (3½ pints) of water a day.

SIGNS THAT YOUR HEART IS UNDER STRESS OR UNHAPPY

A diagonal crease on one or both ear lobes[2]:The face is a great reader of many things and it doesn't stop at emotions. Tales of the diseased body come through the face, the nails, the tongue and the ears, and a creased diagonal line on one or both ear lobes is a predictor of heart disease. The face shows signs of organ weakness or an inflamed system.

Abnormal lunulae on the nail bed: If your lunulae (the white half-moons) on your nails have changed or they have started to appear red in colour, you must consider cardiovascular disease as a cause.

Beau's lines: If there are lines on your nails that run across the nail bed, or if the nail bed looks furrowed and damaged, it could be a sign of a heart attack (myocardial infarction).

Bleeding gums: Healthy gums should be light pink in appearance. Bleeding gums are generally due to a bacterial infection. You can take measures by gargling with salt water to keep the mouth free of bacteria and also by using a soft toothbrush. Bleeding gums can also be a sign of gum disease, so I really would advise checking this out with your dentist.

Sleep apnoea: This is a pause in breathing when you are sleeping and it can happen up to 30 times in a night. It is a condition that disables a restful night's sleep and subconsciously stresses the body's internal organs. It is associated with high blood pressure and arrhythmia of the heart.

Swollen feet and legs: A pooling of liquid in the lower extremities is called oedema and is a sign of heart failure. The fluid build-up is due to a reduced flow out of the heart, causing the blood that is returning to the heart through the veins to back up. This leads to fluid accumulation in the abdomen and lower limbs, as well as congestion.

Sweating: Sweating when there has been no physical exertion is a sign of a heart attack. This happens when the heart does not get enough blood, because if so, the heart doesn't get enough oxygen, which can trigger a heart attack.

Fatigue: If the pumping of the heart starts to reduce you may experience tiredness or fatigue as less blood is available to reach the muscles and the tissues, making you feel weaker.

Hawthorn for the heart

The hawthorn berry has been used for centuries for the heart. Every part of the hawthorn bush – including the flowers, berries, leaves and even the bark – is used to make medicines. Herbalists have identified bioflavonoids, proanthocyanidins and other antioxidants as the active ingredients that make hawthorn so effective. As a medicinal herb it has been used for high blood pressure, atherosclerosis and arrhythmia. Hawthorn also contains the compound quercetin, which has been shown to reduce cholesterol.

Case study

Wounds to the heart

You need to 'Wash That Man Right Out of Your Hair!' That's what I immediately wanted to say to Mimi, and then I wanted to add, 'You need to climb down off that miserable roundabout of /

love me, I hate me, which keeps so many of us tired, dizzy and miserable.'

But of course, that's not my role and every client has their own story that needs to be heard and understood so that I can help them in the way that's right for them. There are so many women like Mimi, who come to me concerned and alarmed about physical manifestations of troubled emotions. And in case you think I sound holier than thou, I know this for a fact because I've been there too. I know our wonderful bodies protect us from so much, until we're ready (or forced) to listen to what we should have heard earlier, but, like Boudicca in full warrior-queen mode, until that point we battle on through the slings and arrows, because it can sometimes seem safer to continue steering that chariot through hell and high water than do something about it!

Some of us let a glass of wine, or several, help. Others use drugs, extreme exercise, lots of sugar, sex or shopping to make us feel better. Anything and everything can become an addiction, and addictions exist because of circumstances such as heart-break, denial, unexploited potential, lost expectation, failure or frustration. Few of us are lucky enough to be free of these in one form or another. Like Polyfilla, we can use what we choose, as a temporary measure, although there's always the risk that something temporary can become permanent. My own Polyfilla was exercise; I shut the door on my emotions and trained my body excessively so as not to allow them any space whatsoever. However, you can only use so much Polyfilla before you need to accept that only a complete re-plastering will do. It is the journey of the re-plastering that has no definitive end; it is up to you and the strength that you find within you to do whatever it takes to get back on the rollercoaster of life. Mimi was dealing with excessive behaviour, overconsumption of food and alcohol, which had forced her weight into the 'I hate my body' zone.

I met Mimi at a point where I could see how her story might play out, but my defined role as a nutrition and lifestyle coach was to support and guide. As Emma Lane, founder of Integrative Health Education, once told me, the most effective therapists and practitioners are those who have experienced life and can call on shared experience without actually sharing. Like many of us, Mimi had been catapulted off the conveyor belt of life when she least expected it and was struggling to climb back on again, so the weight was going up and not coming down. When a person is in chaos, you need to move them slowly but surely away from that chaos and not add to it. A common and frequent mistake is to give the client too much to do, too quickly. If your mind is jumping up and down like a demented monkey, a radical and complicated health plan involving supplements, cooking, exercise and lifestyle change will only add to the confusion, so instead you need to keep it simple and achievable.

My prescription for Mimi at our second session was simply to drink 3 litres (5 pints) of water every day. I recommended she sit down with a cup of tea before going home to chaos and also change which station she got off at, so she could walk the last bit home, taking in new surroundings and allowing her to brain-dump and cultivate calm. My last suggestion, because she'd freely admitted she always fared badly in any confrontation – and that made her miserable – was to remove herself, for the present, from any conflict that she may find at home.

As the months went on I came to realise that Mimi was a complicated and tortured soul. It is often easy to see the way out of the situation you are looking at when it's not your situation to move out of in the first place, so holding back your opinion is paramount.

I gave Mimi my phone number and asked her to send me a picture of herself in the gym every morning, and I would do the same. I wanted her to break the cycle and feel the positive, enhancing benefits that exercise would give her. It was a shared contract, too, so it also got me out of bed each morning and made me run around the park looking for an appropriate spot to take a selfie! We took it in turns to send pictures; me running all puffed out or her in the gym, sometimes with a smile, sometimes without. It worked and her weight started to go in the right direction – down.

I reminded her as she sat in front of me crying or ranting or searching, frustrated and upset, that this was hard work, this was the apprenticeship, this was the part of the painting job that everyone hates. All we want to do is put the paint on the roller and roll away and see that new colour on the wall. No one likes the preparing, the sanding, the covering of the skirting boards and the overalls – that's the stuff dads do. I encourage my clients to do the preparation work so that it only needs to be done once. Or, I say, I can lock you in the bathroom until you've lost the weight, but the problem with starvation is that you learn nothing and the moment you get to the goal weight you pile it back on again and jump back on the emotional rollercoaster of life.

Mimi had a relationship with antidepressants, extreme weight loss and weight gain, so this was not a simple situation of eat less, exercise more, or eat more, exercise less. She was a work in progress because we are all a work in progress, every single one of us. The wounds of the heart play out in many ways, every single day. It's about having the tools to be able to recognise your traits that no longer serve you and thanking them for making you the person you are today. It's a journey that we all learn from.

Today Mimi is at her lightest, she has her ducks in a row and

> feels stronger than ever, with a new job and new enthusiasm.
> It was a difficult journey with a lot of tough love along the way,
> but she took responsibility for her life and I supported her, and
> when she started to veer off the path, I was there to steer her
> back onto it again!

Cardiovascular disease

Cardiovascular disease is one of the most preventable disease states
and more people die prematurely from it than any other disease. It
can occur when the coronary arteries that feed the heart start to get
blocked up over time, resulting in a heart attack. The body does and
can heal itself, and plant-based foods, lean meats, water and lifestyle
choices can de-plaque your arteries and lower your blood pressure.

Nutritional prevention plan for cardiovascular disease

Lifestyle medicine is about preventing chronic disease. It is about
putting in place preventative nutrition and lifestyle plans, thereby
looking after the physiology of your body, and that is the key to living
a long, beautiful, pain-free life. That's the great thing – you can do
something about it! Small changes such as drinking water in the
morning, getting off the sofa and going for a walk instead of watching
TV, walking to work (if you're close enough) and eating foods from the
plan below will help you make a start on the journey to better health.

Time	What to eat for healthy blood vessels
Upon waking	A glass of water and a full body stretch (never start the day with caffeine)
Breakfast	Goldilocks porridge – oats, almond milk, turmeric and raw honey
Mid-morning snack	Mixed fresh berries

Lunch	Chicken stir-fry in lamb's lettuce wraps: stir-fry chicken strips in coconut oil, with ginger and tamari sauce and red/yellow peppers and courgette strips. Stuff into wraps and munch
Mid-afternoon snack	Courgette canapés: sliced raw courgettes topped with nut butter, hummus or olive tapenade
Dinner	Baked cod with sumac spice, wilted spinach and leeks on a bed of buckwheat noodles. Season as you like

Cardiovascular disease is the number one killer of the twenty-first century, but if prescriptions looked like those above, perhaps we would go some way to changing this. Treating the risk factors is not working; we need to get to a preventable prescription system to change and strengthen the physiology in the body so that the body does not become reliant on the drugs but is given the chance to start healing itself and preventing disease.

> *'If you always do what you have always done, you will always get what you have always got.'*
> *- Henry Ford (1863-1947)*

High blood pressure (Hypertension)

A modern-day preventable disease and yet the biggest killer in the Western world, high blood pressure, otherwise known as hypertension, has a lot to answer for. Over five million people are unaware that they have high blood pressure, yet it affects more than one in four adults and is one of the biggest risk factors for premature death and disability in England. High blood pressure can lead to conditions such as heart disease, stroke, vascular dementia and chronic kidney disease.

Blood pressure (BP) is the pressure of circulating blood in the walls of blood vessels, but increased blood pressure, i.e. too much blood in the blood vessels, puts strain on the heart, it can damage the blood vessels that feed the eyes and the kidneys and can cause bleeding in the brain. Hypertension has the ability to cause so many problems in all organ systems of the body that its prevention is multifactorial. BP is usually expressed in terms of the systolic (maximum pressure in one heartbeat) pressure over the diastolic (the minimum pressure in between two heartbeats) and is measured in millimetres of mercury (mmHg). Blood pressure, along with respiratory rate, heart rate, oxygen saturation and body temperature, is one of the vital signs of life-sustaining functions.

Hypertension can come with no symptoms at all, but at the same time high blood pressure can be caused by diet and lifestyle – you may be either too stressed to notice your body falling out of balance or you are being so numbed by processed food and sugar that you don't notice these physiological changes to your body. It is the wear and tear on blood vessels from diet and lifestyle that gives this disease its name as the silent killer.

The best way to identify it is to get your blood pressure checked with your doctor. Hypertensive crisis (usually due to secondary high blood pressure) is defined as a blood pressure reading of 180 or above for the systolic pressure (first number) or 110 or above for the diastolic pressure (second number). Normal resting blood pressure in an adult is 120mmHg/80mmHg.

As there are no obvious ways to identify hypertension other than being tested at your doctor's, it is very important to know what the causes are so that you can take preventative action.

What hypertension might look or feel like to you

Severe headache: We have all had a headache from time to time, and some people suffer from them more than others. Some are alcohol-induced, some are due to dehydration. If you have frequent headaches for which you can't identify the cause, perhaps it's time for a check-up at the doctor's.

Fatigue or confusion: We all get tired from time to time but when the tiredness is overwhelming it would be considered not usual or normal, so, again, it's time for a check-up.

Vision problems: If you are struggling to see things close up, or having blurred vision that may also feel straining on your eyes that is not relieved by any of your usual tried-and-tested tricks, have a check-up.

Anxiety: You may feel not quite yourself and do not understand why. If something feels off then it is better to get checked out by your doctor.

How can I prevent high blood pressure?

Diet and lifestyle: When the pressure in your blood vessels increases you create high blood pressure. There are certain foods that will cause your BP to increase; if the food on your plate has been dyed a funny colour, if the list of ingredients reads like a dissertation, if it doesn't rot and if it causes you to overeat, what you are eating probably isn't real food. So eat food that is fresh and seasonal and colourful. Fresh vegetables, fresh fruits and berries, whole grains, lean meats and fatty fish! Refer to the season chart on pages 317–21.

Smoking and alcohol: Drinking alcohol in moderate amounts, especially red wine, can have lowering effects on blood pressure, but this is not true with overconsumption – which would be more than two glasses of wine a night. Smoking, as we know, has no beneficial effects on anyone's health, only adverse effects.

Stress: Stress in any form – whether it be financial, concerning a relationship, moving house, divorce, a broken bone or an injury – creates tension and puts pressure on the whole body and the blood vessels. Happy, positive thoughts lead to happy positive actions, which leads to normal blood pressure.

Sodium: This is your table salt and you'll have to do more than just refrain from passing the salt cellar – as a starting point, use mineral-rich Celtic sea salt instead. Having said that, it is more to do with the food you are eating, such as takeaways, ready-made meals and pre-cooked foods, as these often contain very high sodium levels, so cutting these out can greatly reduce your salt intake. Read the labels and know your limits; for an average-sized adult, sodium intake should be no more than 6g of salt (2.4g sodium) a day.

Excess weight: Being overweight is a sign of an unhappy body. An overweight body puts stress everywhere: on the musculoskeletal system which holds you up, on the lymphatic system which provides drainage for the body, on the respiratory system which gives you breath, on the circulatory system which makes your blood flow around the body transporting nutrients and life. So if you are overweight, all these systems and more will have to work harder and those blood vessels will feel the strain. By moving and sweating 20 minutes every day you will notice the difference in how you feel and how you look. Unfortunately, a pill will not do this for you. So get up and get out!

Caffeine: If you wake up in the morning and the first thing you think of is a double espresso, you are living with a stressed body and the chances are your day revolves around food, which gives you instant gratification, and caffeine. If it's in the form of an energy drink, stop! – that stuff can do so much damage; equally, if the drink is blue or red, keep a long arm away from it. These drinks are all chemical cocktails that can be associated and linked with hypertension, diabetes and heart palpitations.

Other ways to help prevent high blood pressure
Eat sources of nitric oxide: Nitric oxide is a key messenger in the body and basically opens up your arteries; it allows them to relax

and let more blood flow through them. Viagra works in a similar way; it boosts nitric oxide significantly, which relaxes the arteries and improves the blood flow. Luckily for us humans, we have the ability to make nitric oxide, and beetroot and greens are rich in it, which is essentially why people see sports performance gains when drinking pure beetroot juice (doping with beetroot juice) before exercise. Try to get more Swiss chard, beetroot, basil, lettuce, spring greens, coriander, rocket and rhubarb into your diet. The easiest way to do this would be to make sure you eat a green salad every day.

Take flaxseed: Full of omega 3 fatty acids, which time and time again have been proven to lower blood pressure, flaxseed may protect against atherosclerotic cardiovascular disease by reducing serum cholesterol, improving glucose tolerance and acting as an antioxidant.

Use cardamom: This versatile spice comes from southern India and has been proven to have positive results in lowering blood pressure.

Eat garlic: Well known for its ability to lower blood pressure by causing blood vessels to relax and dilate, allowing blood to flow more freely and reducing blood pressure.

Do exercise: Exercise is always going to be a drug-free approach to lowering or improving anything. Regular physical activity makes your heart stronger. A strong heart can pump more blood with less effort and if your heart can work less to pump, the force on your arteries decreases, lowering your blood pressure. Make sure you stick to the low-impact kind of exercise, such as mat Pilates, swimming, yoga, meditation and country walks. Exercise loves the heart.

Address emotional issues: What is the underlying cause of high blood pressure that you are not addressing? What is boiling up to pressure point without you noticing? Tai-chi is a great meditative practice to calm the body and mind and to encourage you to focus on the breath and movement as one. When you are totally immersed in the moment you are focused on you and you have found inner balance. Having hypertension is a long way off from finding inner balance.

Arteriosclerosis

Arteriosclerosis describes the thickening and hardening of the walls of the arteries, which typically occurs in old age. The condition occurs when plaque builds up on the walls of the arteries, increasing blood pressure and pulse pressure. As the walls thicken they also lose elasticity and harden. It can affect all large- and medium-sized arteries, including the coronary, carotid and cerebral arteries, the aorta and major arteries of the extremities. It is the leading cause of morbidity and mortality in the US and in most developed countries. Damage to a blood vessel wall causes inflammation in the area as well as increased permeability and migration of phagocytes. Phagocytes are cells that protect the body by eating up bacteria, dying or dead cells.

What arteriosclerosis might look or feel like to you

Chest pain or angina pectoris: This can present as a tightening across the chest and a shortness of breath. It can feel as if there is pressure on the heart area which can come in episodes. It is a restriction of blood flow to the heart.

Pain in your leg, arm and anywhere else that has a blocked artery: This pain may increase on walking or moving. Muscle weakness occurs in your legs from lack of circulation.

Fatigue: This is general fatigue that may accompany the other cited symptoms.

Confusion: This occurs if the blockage affects circulation to your brain.

Thrombosis: Complications that can arise from arteriosclerosis include thrombosis, which is an intravascular blood clot remaining in the place where it is formed, or an embolism, which is when an embolus (mobile blood clot) travels through the blood and causes a blockage.

Other ways to help prevent arteriosclerosis

Limit the trans fats in your diet: These bad, man-made fats, such as margarine and shortening, lard, spreadable butters in tubs and vegetable oils, love to clog the arteries. These trans fats cause plaque to build up and increase pressure in the arteries, resulting in high blood pressure. Watch out for reduced-fat labels as they often contain trans fats or hydrogenated fats. When you do use fats, choose good fats – monounsaturated fats such as olive oil and avocados, or polyunsaturated fats found in certain fish, nuts and seeds, which are also good choices for a heart-healthy diet.

Eat more fruit and veg: Eating more fruits and vegetables will undoubtedly save lives, while eating solely fast-foods and processed meats that resemble Play-Doh will kill. Food alone has the power to heal or to poison, and that is a fact. We accept that smoking is a leading cause of lung cancer, we accept that drinking vast amounts of alcohol will cause liver damage, we accept that if we overeat and under-exercise we can put on weight, but what we need to understand and accept, too, is that food has the ability to play its role in pathologies of the organs, by changing the environment they live in. When the environment changes, the beautiful and perfectly shaped happy cells turn into angry cells that want to self-destruct. If your diet consists of more Play-Doh-type food than fruit or vegetables you will create a pressure on the body and pressure on the blood vessels and that can lead to some serious pathologies.

Connect with your heart: The heart chakra is the fourth chakra, full of love, warmth, compassion and joy, and it is located in the centre of the chest at heart level. Being perceptive to our physical sensations within our own heart is a gift that not everyone is sensitive to. The connection between the physical sensations of the body and the emotions that arise has been known for a very long time, but being perceptive to our physical sensations within our own heart is a skill not everyone has. Often the things we cannot see or feel are not understood, and this is true of the physical and emotional manifestations of the organs. Open up to the people around you, practise being open and sharing some personal thoughts or emotions with those you feel safe with and whom you trust. Feel the fear and do it anyway!

Exercise regularly: Taking regular exercise starts a cascade of good things and in turn will improve your health. Regular exercise will not only stabilise or lower blood pressure but also decrease stress, making you feel more energetic. Feeling better persuades us to make better choices with our food and therefore have more positive thoughts. If you're new to exercise, start with a brisk walk in nature and build up to what your body is asking for.

TOP 10 TIPS FOR A HEALTHY HEART

1. **Increase your magnesium intake:** Magnesium is your heart's best friend and through modern-day stress it gets depleted. You can find it in halibut – 75g (3 oz) of white fish would give you 70mg of magnesium; 180g (6 oz) of legumes or beans would give you 120mg; 100g (3½ oz) of dark green leafy vegetables – kale, spinach and chard – or pumpkin seeds would give you 350mg; 100g (3½ oz) of nuts would give you 150mg, and 100g (3½ oz) dark chocolate would give you 295mg.

2. **Crush garlic:** Garlic facilitates the arteries to become less stiff and to remain in better health, preventing or certainly warning of conditions like atherosclerosis and high blood pressure. When eaten raw, garlic is also a potent inhibitor of blood clotting. In one study by Dr Budoff in 2015 at the University of Missouri[3], it was found that taking 2,400mg

of garlic extract a day slowed the total plaque accumulation by 80 per cent, which slowed the progression of atherosclerosis and reversed the early stages of heart disease.

3. **Drink hawthorn tea:** Otherwise known as the gentle heart herb, hawthorn has been taken for centuries for heart health. Hawthorn leaves, flowers and fruits contain certain chemical compounds that increase the flow of blood to the heart muscle as well as providing positive effects for the whole cardiovascular system.

4. **Sweat it out:** There is no better tonic for the heart than to be exercised. Running, power walking, dancing, playing with your kids, the gym, sex, cycling, housework – it is all exercise/movement. If you move, you are exercising, and if you are always changing the gear you move in, i.e. going from fast to slow and vice versa, your body is always having to adapt, which keeps it strong, healthy and efficient.

5. **Devour some dark chocolate (cacao):** Cacao has benefits to the cardiovascular system. Milk chocolate has high amounts of bad fat and refined sugars with little or no benefits to the cardiovascular system; however, organic dark chocolate with 85 per cent cocoa solids can dilate the arteries two hours after eating and improve arterial function. It is also a potent antioxidant. Health tip – do not eat dark chocolate with milk as the oxalic acid blocks the absorption of calcium in the milk.

6. **Love and be loved:** One of the best pieces of advice I heard once was never go to sleep on an argument. Arguments are a waste of time if they are not resolved. They take up too much of your brain power and headspace and then manifest into your thoughts, creating negativity, eventually seeping into the pathomorphology of your tissues. Before you go to sleep, take a piece of paper and write it all down so that you can sleep with a clear mind.

7. **Juice red cabbage:** Red cabbage juice contains lots of omega 3 fatty acids that lower your cholesterol and triglycerides, thus helping to prevent cardiovascular disease and strokes, and lowering blood pressure, too. Sometimes the pathways to your heart get a bit sticky and need some cleaning out, so add a thumbnail of ginger[4]! A shot of cold-pressed

red cabbage and ginger with a touch of apple to make it palatable will open up your arteries and create silky, fluid blood flow to your heart.

8. **Find happiness:** If you do not do what you love or what you want in life you will not find happiness. Ask yourself what you don't want and start from there; make a list or draw a picture of what you want in this beautiful life of yours and start decluttering your life.

9. **Snack on walnuts:** Any more than a handful is too much, so keep your nut habit in check. Walnuts are not only the top nut for a dense anti-oxidant content to protect against cell damage but they are great for the brain, too. A serving of 28g (1oz) of walnuts will keep you satisfied as a compliant health snack more than any other nut. Walnuts are also rich in alpha-linolenic acid, or ALA, which can convert to omega 3s in the body and have been reported to lower total cholesterol and triglycerides in people with high cholesterol levels.

10. **Be still:** Try to practise the fine art and underrated activity of doing nothing! Try relaxing, lying down or walking barefoot. When you stop or take your pace of life down a gear you allow your blood pressure to drop and your heart rate to decrease, which gives your heart a well-needed rest. When you are stressed your body craves high-calorie fatty and sugary foods, which are not beneficial for heart health.

Footnotes

(1) Hartley, L. et al, 'Green and black tea for the primary prevention of cardiovascular disease', *Cochrane Database of Systematic Reviews* (2013).

(2) Bezanis, R., *Diagnostic Face Reading and the Holistic You* (USA, 2010).

(3) Varshney, R., Budoff, M., 'Garlic and Heart Disease', *Journal of Nutrition* (Oxford, 2016).

(4) Bordia, A., Verma, S. K., Srivastava, K. C., 'Effect of ginger (*Zingiber officinale* Roscoe) and fenugreek (*Trigonella foenum-graecum* L.) on blood lipids, blood sugar and platelet aggregation in patients with coronary artery disease', *Prostaglandins, Leukotrienes and Essential Fatty Acids* (Oxford, 1997).

8. THE STOMACH

Anxiety, self-doubt and worry; sympathy and reflection

WHAT DOES MY STOMACH DO AND WHERE DOES IT LIVE?

The function of a pouch is to hold something until the appropriate time for release. In the same way that a mother kangaroo holds its baby joey until it is safe to let it bounce off, the stomach holds your protein and releases it when it has been efficiently broken down into a liquid that is safe to pass through to the duodenum of the small intestine.

Lying on the left side of the upper abdomen, shaped like the letter 'J', is your stomach. The stomach has four parts to it and is an essential organ for digestion.

Inside the stomach and lining its walls is a thick layer of mucus, which stops your stomach digesting itself with the harsh acid inside it, which defends against unwanted bugs and opportunist pathogens that enter your body. This acid is potent, with a pH of 1.5–3.5, and its job is to break down the toughest of the three macronutrients – protein – so there must be an abundant supply. The food slides down the oesophagus, through the lower oesophageal sphincter and drops into the pool of acid like someone whizzing down a water slide into the plunge pool at the bottom. If the plunge pool is empty you may experience a few assaults to the body, but if it's full of water it is a pleasurable experience. Having adequate supplies of HCL is healthy and happens effortlessly; if the acid is in short supply you may experience heartburn, indigestion or an inability to eat rich or protein-based foods.

Facts

- A starfish can turn its stomach inside out.
- When a frog is sick it throws up its stomach first.
- Cows and other 'ruminants', including giraffes, deer and cattle, have four-chambered stomachs which help them digest their plant-based food.
- Seahorses, lungfishes and platypuses have no stomach. Their food goes from the oesophagus straight to the intestines.

Did you know?

In 1868, German doctor Adolf Kussmaul used an endoscope to look inside the stomach of a living person for the first time. Kussmaul employed the talents of a sword swallower who could easily gulp down the 47 x 1.3cm (18½ x ½ inch) instrument that Kussmaul designed.

EMOTIONS OF THE STOMACH

The meridian of the stomach

When the meridian of the stomach is in flow your appetite for food and life is strong. The stomach meridian lies below the eye, to the jawline, then travels around the back, down to the neck, traversing the ribcage and down through the abdomen, along the anterior aspect of the foot, ending at the second toe (face, chest and outer legs). The stomach meridian can affect the stomach, digestive system, vision, sense of taste, menstruation, knees and production of saliva. If the stomach meridian is out of balance you may have general intestinal distress, vomiting, stomach aches, facial paralysis, knee pain, gastritis and indigestion.

Properties of the stomach meridian

Force: Yang (male)

Chakra: Solar plexus – personal power, self-will

Organ body clock: 7–9am

Season: Summer (Indian)

Colour: Yellow

Fragrances: Sweet

Metaphysical lesson: Sympathy and reflection

Emotions of the stomach

It is here in the stomach that all undigested ideas, thoughts, emotions and feelings start to get addressed. Alexithymia is a disorder by which you are unable to recognise or express your feelings. If you are unable to express yourself you are likely to have digestive problems. If this is the case, changing your diet and exercise plan will only go some way to helping and will only ever be short term until the true expression of yourself is dealt with.

Psychoneuroimmunology is the study of the emotions and how they affect different parts of the body. The relationship between mental health and stress is becoming more prevalent, and so too are the pathologies of the specific organs. The energy of the stomach is Yang and the spleen (the place where old red blood cells are recycled) balances this with a Yin energy. The stomach not only digests food but also emotions and experiences, and the stomach, when in balance, is a place of stability and centring, but when out of balance all aspects of your life can feel out of kilter. The stomach holds stress and anxiety and when they are controlled, so too is the health of the stomach.

If the stomach is in balance there is more ability to create nourishing relationships with others and deal with the emotions that those relationships can bring. When the stomach is out of balance you may experience feelings of anxiety, a sense of being unsafe, perhaps entering or staying in co-dependent relationships, and your skin may start to flare up.

THE FOUR BODIES OF THE STOMACH

The spiritual body

In traditional Chinese medicine a balanced stomach represents your ability to have balanced relationships and to face the challenges that life presents you with. The stomach is a Yang energy and so needs movement in order to digest not only food but thoughts, situations and energies. Movement stimulates movement and a strong stomach sets the rest of the body up for optimum health, too.

Action: Try forest bathing. The Japanese call it shinrin-yoku and it has been scientifically proven to improve your health by reducing stress hormones, reducing blood pressure, improving your immune system and increasing your overall feelings of wellbeing.[1] It takes a 30-minute dose of nature to lower your sympathetic nervous system control. Tip: don't take your phone!

The emotional body

Every single emotional state that we as humans experience is reflected in the gut. When the stomach is angry it contracts, produces more acid secretion and more blood has to pump to the stomach to do more work. The anger of the stomach will most likely produce feelings of anxiety and stress, as now the two hormones adrenaline and noradrenaline start to circulate around your body making your skin clammy, and your heart will start to beat faster.

There are lots of things we say that connect our inner thoughts and feelings to parts of our body, such as 'I've got butterflies in my tummy'. The stomach is also referred to as an organ of intuition, as in 'a feeling in my gut', or in terms of bravery and not being able to stomach something or not having the guts to do it.

For some people with sensitive or fragile stomachs, when anxiety strikes you may feel a pain, a stabbing sensation or nausea. Emotions and feelings can sit in the stomach waiting to be digested, much like the way food is held in the stomach before it is absorbed by the rest of the body for energy.

Being mentally healthy plays a hugely important part in addressing digestive health. Happy mind, happy tummy.

Action: Read a book that transports you somewhere else. A fiction book, or even a book from childhood. One of my favourites is *The Wind in the Willows* by Kenneth Grahame, as it always conjures up such colourful imagery and allows my mind to be transported somewhere else for a time.

The nutritional body

The stomach is often referred to as the sea of nourishment because it is responsible for passing the nutrients of the food and fluid that we eat to the rest of the body. It is the first organ to receive nourishment in the form of food and drink.

Food is nourishment and nourishment is love, and love comes through food in a positive or a negative way. Food is seen as a reward, a treat; we can be in love with food, use it for survival and as a comfort. Food is an excellent mimic for lost love and opportunity and it never answers back. When we have lost a certain desire, food is first in line to step in and ease the blow and fill the gaping hole of loneliness, grief, death and emptiness. Just as you cannot digest certain foods, the same can be said of not being able to digest certain emotions, and this is when your stomach starts talking to you. So if you feel like you have knots in your stomach, it's time to start paying attention.

Action: Avoid foods that are hard to break down and lack nutritional integrity, such as processed foods and refined sugars. Foods that make you happy and feed your brain will come from the soil, not the packet; from the sea and not from a farmed lake; from the fields and not from caged pens; from the seasons (see chart on pages 317–21) and not from GM factories. The choices you make with your food ultimately make up the balance of your emotions, so eat wisely.

The physical body

Staying active gives your mind distractions, and distractions provide you with a mental break that can reduce future anxiety symptoms. One issue for people with anxiety is inactivity. Moving and staying physically active are extremely important for mental health; it improves hormone function and neurotransmitter production and is a great way to manage anxiety. Visceral manipulation is a gentle manual therapy that helps your body to release restrictions and unhealthy compensations which cause pain and dysfunction. VM helps calm GI inflammation and stimulate nerve connections. The only exception to this would be when the client was experiencing pain or abdominal swelling. Acupuncture, acupressure and reiki are all useful alternatives for creating calm and decreasing stress and anxiety.

Start the day with this piston breathing exercise:

Action: Piston breathing is an ancient technique that increases oxygen supply to the body and all its organs. A great way to shift your mood if you are feeling anxious or stressed.

Standing in a relaxed posture, inhale deeply, allowing your belly to expand.

Exhale forcefully through your nose. If you can't breathe through your nose, exhale through your mouth while pursing your lips like a trumpet player.

Inhale again slowly, repeat, and build up to 100 exhalation pulses.

HOW TO KEEP YOUR STOMACH HAPPY

Your stomach will love you if you eat an array of healing foods. Eating well is not only a consideration for your personal health, being irresponsible for your health has a price to pay on the world you live in. Good eating practices put less stress and pressure not only on your body, mind and soul but also on the environment. By starting with ourselves we all contribute to looking after this beautiful world we live in. Try to purchase food from organic markets to ensure the food is fresh and seasonal, rather than in packets from the supermarket, which will also help to decrease your use of plastics and your carbon footprint.

Nutritional plan for a healthy stomach

How to maintain optimum digestion and create a good relationship with food.

Dos	Why	Outcome / result / response
Think about what you want to eat to whet your appetite	This stimulates your saliva glands which produce salivary amylase to help break down your food	Creates a cephalic response which is essential for digestion
Sit down to eat at a table and take time to eat three times a day, allowing 20–30 minutes for each meal	Our most enjoyed pastime must take place within a relaxed parasympathetic state for optimum digestion	Creates a parasympathetic response needed for optimum digestion, absorption and elimination of food

Take a digestive enzyme or 1 tablespoon of apple cider vinegar 10 minutes before food	Helps further breakdown of the food for digestion and absorption of food	Creates optimum digestion and improves IBS symptoms, such as bloating and gas
Drink water 10 minutes before you eat and sip throughout your meal	Too much water can deplete your digestive enzymes which impairs digestion	Creates optimum digestion and reduces bloating
Don't watch TV or read the newspaper while eating	These actions create stressful environments	Creates a stress response and activates the sympathetic nervous system which can impair digestion in the stomach
Do not rush	Eating is about healing so take your time and relax – those emails will still be there in 20 minutes' time	Creates impaired digestion, heartburn and indigestion

Cabbage juice for the stomach

Juicing raw cabbages has been clinically proven to improve conditions such as peptic ulcers of the stomach.[2] L-glutamine is an amino acid that is needed for protein synthesis and helps regenerate cell repair for the intestinal lining. It is the main nutrient found in cabbages.

Supplements to support the function of the stomach

These supplements help the stomach's function when it is running out of the necessary acids, enzymes and co-factors to further break food down for absorption in the small intestines.

Plant-based digestive enzymes: Plant-based enzymes are able to work in the acidic environment of the stomach and the neutral environment of the intestines, whereas animal proteins cannot. They contain natural proteins that will help break down your food into smaller, more digestible particles and increase absorption for your food, too.

Multivitamin with copper: Multivitamins don't often have copper in them, which is essential for the uptake of zinc.

Vitamin B12: The stomach produces intrinsic factor (see page 256) which is essential for the absorption of B12 in the stomach as well as for protein breakdown. A B12 deficiency causes your immune system to attack the cells in your stomach that produce intrinsic factor, which can increase the risk of pernicious anaemia.

This can be taken as an intracellular injection if levels get too low, or as a tablet or drops under the tongue. It is essential, meaning your body doesn't make it, so you must ingest it through food such as meat, eggs and cheese.

Zinc carnosine: Zinc is essential for the production of hydrochloric acid, made by the chief cells of the stomach, which is responsible for denaturing protein for absorption as well as having a direct anti-inflammatory effect on the stomach. Pumpkin seeds, as well as most red meat and poultry which have the highest levels of zinc, are good sources. Making sure your diet is also high in vitamin C, E, B6 and magnesium increases your absorption of zinc.

Aloe vera: This is an amazing plant with valuable medicinal properties that aid in healing a variety of ailments. Aloe is a very soothing plant for the stomach when you are experiencing bloating, nausea or just an upset stomach.

SIGNS THAT YOUR STOMACH IS UNHAPPY

Acid reflux/heartburn: This is acid that is forced out of the stomach via the lower oesophageal sphincter and into the oesophagus, which can happen after eating food or at night when lying down. This is usually a case of too little acid, not too much. So if you are taking antacids because you have symptoms of acid reflux, you could well be depleting the already depleted store of HLC.

Nausea: This can often be experienced when there is a lack of HCL in the stomach, especially when eating rich or high-protein foods.

Constipation: If the body is not breaking down the food it is not absorbing it and it will also not be eliminating it.

Pain in your sternum: This is due to acid being in the wrong place, not necessarily having too much of it. If the lower oesophageal sphincter is loose this can give rise to acid leaking into the oesophagus, causing pain in the sternum.

Vomiting: This can be a sign of an ulcer. An ulcer in the stomach is called a peptic ulcer, while an ulcer in the small intestine is called a duodenal ulcer.

POST-PRANDIAL SOMNOLENCE – OR FOOD COMA

If you ever find someone slumped across the sofa looking as if they can't move or muster a conversation, communicating only with grunts and gesticulations, you can be sure they have slipped into a food coma. This is medically referred to as post-prandial somnolence, but I like the good old-fashioned food coma: it says what it does on the tin. Luckily for humans, overeating and greed are universal traits so the symptoms are universally recognised and therefore treatment is too. Leave the client to sleep it off, removing all surrounding plates of food in case they wake and eat!

Doing anything to excess – exercise, alcohol, food and shopping – will reduce your body's stores and you will feel depleted; a food coma is no exception. I've seen the effects first-hand on many occasions! Once, on my birthday, my friends and I went to an Italian restaurant. As a protein type I ordered steak, as did my good friend Hulya. However, the rest of the crew excitedly tucked into a plate full of dough with toppings – otherwise known as pizza – and with the champagne lining their stomachs, on top of the antipasti and vegetables, there was no way out, the food coma had reached out its claw and sucked them all in. The conversation was starting to fade, the eyes were flickering and they were all bloated, even my friend Nick, who usually bounces from the walls with energy, was flagging. The only thing that could save us all now was an espresso martini, so that's what we did. Within minutes they were back to their normal excited selves, although for the most part I don't recommend this!

Mastication, or chewing, is an essential part of digestion and the one that most people leave out. I don't know why people try to swallow large amounts of food down an exceptionally narrow hollow, causing heartburn and pain. Why don't we learn? When you chew your food you are breaking it down to a liquid so that it can easily pass through the stomach into the small intestines, where it is absorbed and used for energy.

When you start eating, blood begins to be diverted away from skeletal muscle to aid digestion. It is essential to get the nutrients for the food you eat over into the bloodstream for nutrient uptake. The greater the quantity of food you eat; the more dense the carbohydrates; the more food with tryptophan (a neurotransmitter responsible for mood and serotonin production) in it; and the higher the GI (glycaemic index) of the food will all contribute to the depth and length of the food coma you will fall into.

Hormonal changes caused by the glucose (the sugar, the energy) you eat temporarily send you to sleep. To make sure your day is not plagued by a chemically induced sleep you can eat smaller meals, take your time to chew your food and make sure that the food you eat has a low GI score, so that you are not cranking out insulin every time you eat.

Partial digestion then takes place in the stomach, and muscles in the stomach churn the food to break it down. Hydrochloric acid is released here, which assists in the chemical breakdown of the food – similar to using washing-up liquid to break down the grease on a pan. So, as you can see, overloading the stomach – especially when you don't have the agents to help break down the food – can leave you heading for a catnap on the sofa. So eat small, be relaxed and chew. Chewing is also great exercise to keep your face muscles fit and firm!

PATHOLOGIES OF THE STOMACH

Helicobacter pylori

Helicobacter pylori (H. pylori) is a bacteria that is found on the wall of the stomach and is thought to affect more than half of the world's population. H. pylori has been evolving with human beings for well over 50,000 years, since they migrated out of Africa. The infection has been identified as a Group 1 carcinogen by the World Health Organization. The medical profession overlooks the majority of gastrointestinal dysfunctions and H. pylori is no exception.

The majority of people who are infected with H. pylori have an anxiety status that follows them around like a shadow. Scientists have even attributed ulcers in the stomach to an overgrowth of H. pylori. The overgrowth is seen more often in people with heightened anxiety, as it is thought the problem may result from the ongoing chronic stress that has undermined the immune system response in the digestive tract, which makes the stomach lining more permeable to the bacteria. Studies have shown that people who have to deal with significant stress on a day-to-day basis have an increased incidence of ulcers, not least because people with stomach issues have tendencies to have an intense need to feel supported in life and in everything they do. By wanting to impress all the time, the stomach takes centre stage.

What H. pylori might look or feel like to you

Stomach pain: You may experience any of the following symptoms, such as bloating, nausea, gas, diarrhoea and constipation, because H. pylori interferes with your stomach acid so you can't digest food properly.

Heartburn or acid reflux: These may be frequent occurrences, or even infrequent.

Low energy: If you feel your energy level has changed – if you are getting afternoon slumps or are struggling to find the energy for exercise – then it might be worth investigating. A H. pylori infection creates stress on the body, depletes your energy and your body's ability to digest and use the food you eat for energy.

Feeling the blues and anxiety: Serotonin is made in a healthy digestive system, and this is your happy hormone. Any disruption to this system can deplete serotonin levels, which alters your mood.

Vomiting: This can happen when an ulcer is present, which causes scarring and swelling, in turn causing a narrowing of the duodenum and obstruction of gastric production.

Testing is inconclusive and the treatment is relatively expensive and long term, so the infection is often left alone. However, some carriers of this infection are completely asymptomatic, meaning they have no symptoms at all. However, keep an eye out for any red flags. If you see black stools or blood or mucus in the stools, seek immediate advice from your doctor.

THE IMPORTANCE OF B12 AND INTRINSIC FACTOR

Helicobacter pylori infection can deplete B12 levels which can attribute to the reason you feel tired, fatigued or depressed.

B12 is required to make red blood cells which transport oxygen around the body. It is important to remember that fatigue is not exclusive to a B12 deficiency but it is part of the picture. Without oxygen getting into the cells it doesn't matter how much you sleep, you will still feel fatigued. Signs that you might be deficient in B12 would be feeling sluggish and weak as well as tired, also anxious, dizzy and forgetful. Your hair may be dry, as would your skin be, and you might have dry cuticles on your nails and be missing the little half-moons on your nails known as lunulae.

Intrinsic factor (IF), also known as gastric intrinsic factor (GIF), is a glycoprotein produced by the parietal cells of the stomach. It is necessary for the absorption of vitamin B12 (cobalamin) later on in the small intestine. In some clients *H. pylori* creates an immune reaction against the parietal cells of the stomach. It is these cells that secrete hydrochloric acid and intrinsic factor into the stomach, both essential for assisting in the breakdown of food and the release of vitamins and minerals for the body to absorb in the duodenum. So if you have *H. pylori* it may be causing B12 to be depleted, low stomach acid levels and decreased intrinsic factor – which explains why you feel anxious, tired and depressed.

Case study

The problem with Helicobacter pylori
By Dr Natalie Greenwold

'Phoebe has had abdominal pains and bloating since the age of 12. She is now 19. Her troubles started following two concomitant episodes of gastroenteritis, the first of which was picked up when our housekeeper returned from the Philippines, unwell with severe diarrhoea.

The pains were left-sided and located in her upper abdomen and she started to have intermittent sharp spasms that would pass only on lying down. The pains, once subsided, would result in extreme tiredness.

Phoebe's general health was good and she was thriving; however, as time went on these symptoms were interfering increasingly with her normal life. She started to take time off school quite regularly, unable to get through the day because of the pain. The tiredness was very stressful as the demands at school increased and on occasion a very bad symptom day would coincide with important exams.

Phoebe attended appointments with paediatricians and gastroenterologists over the years. Her tests were normal apart from a low vitamin D level. Gliadin tests and tests for inflammatory bowel disease came back negative. Her stool culture was also reported to be normal. A diagnosis of IBS was made and Phoebe was advised to eliminate wheat from her diet as well as fish – both of which had seemed to bring on symptoms. She was referred for CBT and self-hypnosis to help her manage the pain. Phoebe's father died suddenly when she was six years old and it was felt that her pains may in part be attributable to grief.

Following four years of psychological support Phoebe's abdominal discomfort remained unchanged. She learnt to make space for her symptoms, developed coping strategies and stuck religiously to her gluten-free diet; however, the unpredictable 'bad days' and low energy with a perceived reduced immunity to viral infections remained a continued and depressing problem.

We came across Hannah by recommendation. Phoebe asked me to join her at the appointment. I am a medical doctor. It is true to say that while we attended a number of appointments to help Phoebe before going to see Hannah I was feeling increasingly frustrated on her behalf that nothing really impacted on her quite debilitating symptoms in any meaningful way.

Hannah took a very careful and detailed history from Phoebe; I was impressed by how attentively she listened to her story. She instantly took note of the original attacks of gastroenteritis and explained that a detailed examination of the stool collected under specific conditions was necessary as a chronic pathogen was most likely. I was so relieved to hear this as I had myself suspected this all along and yet the routine stool tests had always come back negative.

We are currently under Hannah's care and feel most grateful to have found support and help for Phoebe, who, while having had a significant emotional burden through the early death of her father, clearly also had abdominal pathology which had never been addressed seriously up until this point. The bowel when dysfunctional may not be diseased and as such is dismissed by traditional medicine with the heart-sink diagnosis of IBS; however, quality of life is massively eroded for sufferers and there is a clear gap in medical provision for people like Phoebe. An integrative approach to their care is much needed and I am confident that great progress can yet be achieved in this domain.

We wanted to share our story to help others and support the quest among health professionals like Hannah to whom we are most grateful.'

I had suspected *H. pylori* in our first meeting, so I started Phoebe on a gastro protocol to improve her digestive capabilities and made some changes to her diet, increasing protein (low purine) because as someone who had been vegetarian, although she did eat fish for the last 10 years, she found that meat protein was hard to digest. This made sense with my *H. pylori* suspicions. Everything was falling into place.

There is often a point when an incident, a holiday, a trauma or an illness starts to fit in with the last time they felt well. This is not always the case but if I listen carefully to what is being said I find I am able to figure out what is going on. There was definitely emotional stress with Phoebe, which was manifesting itself in the stomach. You could say the stomach digests new ideas and beliefs, therefore when the stomach starts to play up with symptoms, you can't digest anymore. You may not be aware of this at all and that would be fairly normal, but on a subconscious level our stomach plays up when adjusting to something new – a thought, belief or new way of life that is hard to assimilate/digest.

Today Phoebe is in a much better place. Her fatigue has lifted, she has lost half a stone, and she is feeling much, much better. There is still some way to go, though, and the length of the journey is the one thing we just cannot predict.

Ways to prevent H. pylori

B12 and intrinsic factor: *H. pylori* can cause a vitamin B12 deficiency which can be one of the causes for clients feeling anxious or depressed. Supplementing with B12 will help improve mood and intrinsic factor is needed for the efficient absorption of B12.

Garlic[3] broth: Garlic is an allium vegetable and is a wonderful antimicrobial to use in the treatment for infections of the stomach such as *Helicobacter pylori*. Studies also show that the use of garlic has decreased the risk of gastric cancer.

Probiotics: A probiotic will help the colonisation of good bacteria and create a healthy environment in the body, which assists with treating H. *pylori,* especially if you have taken antibiotics to eradicate this bacteria.

Matula tea: Matula tea is the best remedy for the eradication of H. *pylori.* The conventional route is triple x therapy – three rounds of antibiotics – which is not something I would advise. If the integrity of the GIT is weak the antibiotics can leave you with more problems. Matula tea is natural, herbal, energetic and potent.

Cranberry juice: Cranberries often spring to mind when a urinary tract infection occurs – or around Christmas time! But these are not the only reasons to be aware of this impressive little berry. High in antioxidant levels, they can also protect you from free radicals in the environment around you, like pollution, as well as inflammation from inside your body caused by processed foods or too much refined sugar. They have more recently been found to have a positive impact on your gut microbiota[4] – anything we can do for a gorgeous gut is something we'll definitely queue up for!

Broccoli sprouts/juice: A study published in *Digestive Diseases and Science* in 2004 found that eating broccoli sprouts twice daily stopped the H. *pylori.* Seven of the nine subjects who took part tested negative immediately after the trial, with six remaining negative when later tested on day 35.[5]

Practise good breathing: It may sound very simple but an inverted breathing pattern can cause problems in the digestive tract, as it immediately recognises this breathing pattern as a stress response. By using muscles in the neck and head, such as the scalenes, upper trapezius and the sternocleidomastoid, the body avoids the diaphragm and adopts an inverted breathing pattern. This can also lead to GERD (gastroesophageal reflux disease – see below) which can be rectified by seeing a physio, visceral manipulator or neuromuscular therapist.

Heal emotional disorders: To combat the emotional disorders that can be exacerbated by H. pylori infection, you need to follow a healing practice which manages universal energy that can be channelled through the hands. The approach I use is one that is considered to be a good alternative for victims of stress and anxiety, and it is also useful for treating depression and other emotional disorders.

Sleep well: Your body needs to rest. Sleep helps you repair yourself and a lack of sleep will make you more sensitive to the effects of stress.

Follow relaxation techniques: Breathing exercises can lead to relaxation. This state helps mitigate pain, if you have any. Yoga can really help with this.

Try therapy: Cognitive behavioural therapy (CBT) is key for changing the way you think, and for feeling better. This is very helpful if you're feeling anxious or stressed. It also helps to develop adaptive abilities, and to improve relationships.

Gastroesophageal reflux disease (GERD): Heartburn

Gastroesophageal disease is a condition in which the stomach acids rise up the oesophageal passage from the stomach causing a sensation of heartburn – it can sometimes travel up your throat and be painful. Heartburn and peptic ulcers are both common symptoms.

After food passes through your oesophagus into your stomach, a muscular valve called the lower oesophageal sphincter (LES) closes to prevent food or acid going back up. Sphincters are like gatekeepers; they say what goes in and what goes out. If the LES relaxes it can allow acid back up your oesophagus from your stomach – which is known as reflux.

What GERD may look or feel like to you

Hypochlorhydria: Hypochlorhydria arises when the acid in the stomach gets too low. An acidic environment is essential for the digestion of protein, to kill bacteria, to allow the stomach to empty and clear, and for the absorption of micronutrients. HCL levels all deplete as we get older and some people are more prone to having low HCL than others because of stress.

When any of these symptoms (indigestion, belching, weak, peeling and cracked fingernails, nausea after taking a herbal supplement and iron deficiency) are present it can and often does lead to GERD, B12 or iron deficiency (anaemia), IBS symptoms or candida. However, because these symptoms are often mistaken for too much acid being present, the normal course of action may be to take a self-medicated course of antacids to neutralise the acid and resolve the discomfort of indigestion or heartburn. This might involve taking PPIs (proton pump inhibitors – medicines that reduce the acid) and sometimes even surgical measures.

Hiatus hernia: A protrusion of the upper stomach into the thorax. This can present due to either a tear in the diaphragm or the thorax.

Often this can be caused by physical reasons such as heavy lifting, smoking, straining with constipation or a frequent cough or sneeze.

Peptic ulcers: These are single or multiple open sores affecting the mucous membranes of the stomach lining and/or the lining of the intestines. Ulcers are usually caused when the digestive lining becomes thinner and less able to withstand the effects of the digestive juices.

Rosacea[6]: This is a common sign of low hydrochloric acid levels. It starts with a flushing of the face, resembling and often being referred to as a butterfly flush.

Rheumatoid arthritis[7]: An auto-immune disease affecting the joints of the body. Low levels of HCL are often found in clients with this disease.

Treatment plan for GERD

Physical	Lifestyle changes	Nutritional	Supplements to help
Lose weight	Avoid emotional eating	Improve digestion	**Aloe vera juice:** The aloe plant naturally reduces inflammation. Look for a brand that has removed the laxative component!
Visceral manipulation – downward pressure therapy	Let go of your biggest fear that is driving you, through therapy, such as CBT	Improve constipation	**Probiotics:** You must reinoculate your gut with a variety of different microorganisms. All bacteria have an enormous influence on your digestion, detoxification and the immune system. *Lactobacillus acidophilus* reduces gastric distention

Sleep with head raised	Spring-clean your house, bedroom, office, kitchen, etc.	Test for food intolerances/ allergies	**Chamomile tea:** The flowers of the plant are the best to get the therapeutic dosage for a soothing treatment. Just add hot water and steep for 2–3 minutes to allow the therapeutic properties to infuse
Improve posture	Get to bed for 10.30pm and optimise sleep	Drink water and jump up and down for 1–2 minutes	**Slippery elm:** This is a supplement that coats the mucosal lining of all linings in the body, containing antioxidants that reduce inflammatory conditions. This helps increase mucus secretion, which protects your gastro-intestinal tract against ulcers and excess acidity
	Mantra: I breathe freely and fully. I am safe. I trust the process of life		

Top tip:

Bicarbonate of soda: This is a good trick for an emergency if you are in pain. Take 1 teaspoon of bicarbonate of soda in a 225ml (8fl oz) glass of water. It may help ease the burning as it will neutralise the stomach acid.

Other ways to help alleviate GERD

Take control of your emotions: The stomach and the brain are in constant flux with emotions. The stomach can be a little ball of anxiety and you have to be able to understand that the anxiety is stemming from the emotions. Learning to be calm and how to ground yourself will help regulate the levels of emotions and anxiety. Find a patch of grass and take off your socks and shoes and walk up and down for 10 minutes, feeling your connection to the Earth.

Move slowly: We can often move at such a fast pace that we forget to stop. If the body is feeling wired and tired, take some rest from exercise. Walk more and relax more. Spend some time barefoot on the grass and feel the ground under the weight of your body.

Avoid foods that can trigger GERD: Alcohol, caffeine, citrus fruits, chocolate and mint, tomatoes, spices, fatty foods, fizzy drinks and refined sugar foods all relax the oesophageal sphincter.

Invivo Clinical – why this is the MOT of your health

I use the GI-MAP test with the majority of clients who come to see me as they predominantly have issues that originate in the stomach and/or the gastrointestinal tract.

The Gastrointestinal Microbial Assay Plus (GI-MAP) was designed by Invivo Cllinical to assess a client's microbiome from a single stool sample, with particular attention to microbes that may be disturbing normal microbial balance and may contribute to perturbations in the gastrointestinal flora or illness. From this test you see a comprehensive collection of microbial targets as well as immune and digestive markers. It screens for pathogenic bacteria, commensal bacteria, opportunistic pathogens, fungi, viruses, and parasites. It primarily uses multiplex, automated, DNA analysis to give integrative and functional assessments of the gastrointestinal microbiome.

GET HUNGRY

There is one last thing I want to impress upon you before we head off to the intestines, and that is the benefits of feeling hungry. Being hungry and having periods of fasting carry many health benefits for the body.

We hear and say the phrase 'I'm hungry' quite a lot, but most of the time we don't actually mean it. However, when we do say it, all that has really happened is food has been completely emptied out of the stomach. Food passes out of your stomach into the duodenum and it can sometimes make a few gurgling noises which we associate with hunger, and of course you may well be hungry. However, hunger as we experience it will be vastly different from the way other cultures in history and in various places around the world today experience it. It is also something we will most likely be fortunate never to truly experience in our lifetime.

Overeating puts a huge pressure on our digestive system but also on our organs, because if this extra food is not used for energy and is instead stored it turns to visceral fat, which lies like a duck-down duvet around our organs, causing pressure. The body can survive and function on much less than we eat as a nation and as an individual because it carries energy stores around with it all day. Remember that a human body can survive without food for up to three weeks. Mahatma Gandhi survived for 21 days without food, but that was Gandhi proving yet again that what you put your mind to you can achieve.

So perhaps we can take a little bit of Gandhi's willpower and eat a little less, then we would be more energy efficient.

Having a juice day or a liquid day is an equally good thing to do to give your digestive system a rest. It is often overloaded, over-packed and overworked on a regular basis, which is why giving it a rest with a fast day can be beneficial and boost your microbiota, too!

My new favourite word is 'borborygmi', which is the result of stomach rumblings in the small intestines, gurglings we associate with hunger. They're due to normal digestion as food, fluid and gases pass through your gastrointestinal tract. When the tract is empty, however, borborygmi are louder because there's nothing in there to muffle the sound. The muscles in the stomach still contract even though the food has been emptied into the small intestines, and the brain then signals to the stomach that there is no food and the growling noises start.

TOP 10 TIPS FOR A HEALTHY STOMACH

1. **Favour your flavonoids:** Increase your intake of berries. Blueberries, strawberries and raspberries are all full of antioxidants and flavonoids which reduce the effects of free radicals that inhibit the growth of bacteria.

2. **Be cautious taking antacids:** Antacids are one of the biggest-selling drugs of all time and work by decreasing the amount of acid in your stomach or neutralising it. They do this because the antacids are bases which have the opposite effect of acids. They can be addictive and can cause stomach acid to deplete; overuse of antacids can cause the stomach to become alkaline.

3. **Eliminate food sensitivities:** Most food sensitivities are the result of proteins that do not get broken down completely and therefore enter the bloodstream as allergens. Protease is an enzyme that is responsible for breaking down proteins, and stomach acid also plays a major role. Pepsin is the stomach's protein acid, and when the acid in the stomach is compromised, so too is pepsin, which means incomplete breakdown of proteins contributing to food allergies.

4. **Look after your sphincters:** Especially your lower oesophageal sphincter. There are certain foods that trigger the loosening of the

LES – chilli, chocolate, peppermint, citrus, tomatoes and alcohol may all be problematic.

5. **Cut out processed food:** Food that is fast, such as pizza, paninis, cakes, biscuits, packaged meats, cheesy chips, takeaways, etc., is going to play havoc in your stomach because of all the chemicals, E numbers, preservatives and sugars that have been added to them to make them taste good and last longer. Your stomach doesn't always recognise these pesticides and chemicals, so it can often struggle to break them down for digestion, putting strain on your digestive system.

6. **Get into your bitters:** Bitters stimulate digestive secretions that help you break down your food, such as Swedish bitters, which you can take 20 minutes before you eat to stimulate the release of the digestive enzymes, to help you digest your food. Digestive bitters also tap into the body's lingual-neuro response that occurs when you taste something bitter. The bitter taste stimulates increased stomach acid production, as well as other digestive juices. Always follow the dosing directions on the bottle.

7. **Drink your food:** Mastication or chewing is the first point of digestion and if you eat your food too quickly, with barely any time being taken for chewing, you strain the acid in your stomach that is needed to break it down. Next time you chew, chew your food until it is liquid; it may not feel liquid but it's now in an absorbable form that your body can assimilate and use properly in the body. You are what you absorb.

8. **HCL supplementation:** While using bitters, lemon and apple cider vinegar will all help, you may need something stronger to bring stomach acid back into balance. Using a betaine HCL supplementation will help the stomach to produce its own levels of HCL.

9. **Boil your bones:** If you are struggling with low stomach acid you will also be deficient in protein, as you require acid to break down the protein. Taking in protein in a digestible form will help, such as gelatin and bone broth (see page 81).

10. **Increase foods that contain B12:** If there are low stomach acids the

absorption of B12 is disrupted and you can either take the supplement in liquid or spray form and/or eat foods high in purines, such as sardines, beef, liver, salmon and eggs.

Footnotes

(1) Hansen, M., Jones, R., Tocchini, K., 'Shinrin-Yoku (Forest Bathing) and Nature Therapy: A State-of-the-Art Review', *International Journal of Environmental Research and Public Health* (Basel, 2017).

(2) Cheney, G., 'Rapid Healing of Peptic Ulcers in Patients Receiving Fresh Cabbage Juice', *California Medicine* (California, 1949).

(3) Jonkers, D. et al, 'Antibacterial effect of garlic and omeprazole on *Helicobacter pylori*', *Journal of Antimicrobial Chemotherapy* (1999).

(4) Dinh, J. et al, 'Cranberry Extract Standardized for Proanthocyanidins Promotes the Immune Response of *Caenorhabditis elegans* to *Vibrio cholerae* through the p38 MAPK Pathway and HSF-1', *PLOS One* (California, 2014).

(5) Galam, M.V., Kishan A.A., Silverman A.L., 'Oral broccoli sprouts for the treatment of *Helicobacter pylori* infection: a preliminary report', *Digestive Diseases and Sciences* (2004).

(6) Epstein, N., Susnow, D., 'Acne rosacea with particular reference to gastric secretion', *California and Western Medicine* (San Francisco, 1931).

(7) Miura, Y. et al, 'Gastroesophageal reflux disease in clients with rheumatoid arthritis', *Modern Rheumatology* (Japan, 2014).

9. THE GASTROINTESTINAL TRACT

Depression, sadness, the blues

The gastrointestinal system is a long and winding road housed between the mouth and the anus. Chemical reactions take place here to break down the food you eat and the liquid you drink into smaller particles to be absorbed into the bloodstream and to be used as energy by you.

When ill health arises, the gut is the first place that I look for answers. Our gut takes on wear and tear from the stresses of life. How we feel plays the most important part in how we eat, and how we feel depends largely on the amount of stress we have in our lives. Eating is the most emotional thing that we, as humans, do – sometimes seven or more times a day – and the food we eat or don't eat makes up the health of the gut.

It is said that 'you are what you eat' and, more recently, 'you are what you don't absorb!' But I say a more accurate description would be 'you are what you don't excrete'. Flashback to the Gillian McKeith days when she was scraping around in plastic boxes full of poo, shouting at mortified, overweight souls who probably wished they'd read the contract small print as their poo became household viewing.

Until Gillian McKeith came along, poo was a subject as taboo as sex, especially in the UK. Just as sex is certainly never easy to discuss, your bowels and their regularity take much of the same awkward tone. To help me with my clients, I have two charts – the Bristol Stool Chart and one from Paul Chek's book *How to Eat, Move and Be Healthy*[1] – which give names and faces to all the potential states of the bowel and consistency of stools in outfits. It is called the Poopy Policeman line-up.

A lot of people do not know what their bowels look like, or how often they go. Being regular by whose standards? I remember a lady once proudly telling me of her regularity of bowel movements; it was only when I asked her what regular was that we discovered that she was chronically constipated. Twice a week is regular if that's what you do every week, but it's not normal. The bowel should move roughly 30 centimetres (12 inches) of faeces a day, preferably three times a day, an hour or so after every meal. That's optimum regularity and what we should be striving for! So if you are moving your bowels once every three days and you've been told this is normal – it isn't. This scenario is becoming more and more common, but in fact a frequency this low indicates severe faecal impaction and can lead to chronic constipation and slow transit disorders, and it is these conditions that will precede diverticular disease, polyposis, haemorrhoids and colorectal cancer.

Facts:

- The GIT is approximately 9 metres (30 feet) long and its surface area could cover a tennis court.[2]
- The GIT runs from the mouth to the anus.
- Food doesn't need gravity to get to your stomach.
- Your saliva houses your digestive enzymes.
- Much of the digestion process happens in your mouth.

A BIT MORE ANATOMY

The gastrointestinal tract runs from your mouth to your anus. It is a complicated tract with lots of processes all working together to ensure that you chew, digest, absorb, assimilate and eliminate your food for energy. To make sure this happens in the most efficient way, a few factors must be taken into consideration.

The small intestines

The pyloric sphincter is a band of smooth muscle connecting the pylorus of the stomach and the duodenum of the small intestines. The small intestine is the most convoluted part of the intestinal tract, absorbing most of the nutrients from the food we eat. The small intestines are roughly 5 metres (16 feet) long and can be separated into three parts: the duodenum connects to the pyloric sphincter of the stomach and is the shortest section of the small intestine (SI), at about 25 centimetres (10 inches) in length. Here, partially digested food called chyme comes from the stomach and is mixed with bile from the gallbladder and gastric juices from the pancreas to complete the digestion in the duodenum. The duodenum connects to the jejunum where all the nutrients are absorbed in a space of 90 centimetres (35 inches). The jejunum connects to the final section of the SI – the ileum – via the ileocaecal sphincter, to empty into the large intestines. The ileum is roughly 1.8 metres (6 feet) long and is where more absorption of nutrients takes place, just in case the jejunum missed them!

The small intestine measures 2.5 centimetres (1 inch) in diameter, which is half the width of the large intestine, and is made up of four layers of tissue which together act like an accordion, folding and opening to create more and more surface area where the absorption of nutrients can take place.

Also in the SI are villi, finger-like projections that absorb the nutrients and allow them to cross over into the bloodstream. The villi further increase the surface area for digestion, as each square inch of mucosa contains around 20,000 villi, so a lot of absorption can happen. On the top of the villi are microvilli, which again further increase the surface area, maximising nutrient and vitamin absorption.

The large intestine

The large intestine measures about 1.5 metres (5 feet) in length and 6–7 centimetres (2–3 inches) in diameter in the living body but becomes much larger postmortem as the smooth muscle tissue of the intestinal wall relaxes.

The job of the large intestine is to absorb water from the remaining indigestible food matter and transit the now-useless waste material from the body. The process that facilitates this is called peristalsis and can take around 36 hours. First, liquid and salt is removed from the waste as it passes through the colon, then the waste makes its way to the sigmoid colon, where it is stored. Once or twice a day, when the body is ready for a bowel movement, the waste is dumped into the rectum until your body decides it's time to excrete it.

Peristalsis is the contraction and relaxation of the stomach muscles to physically break down food and propel it forward through the gastrointestinal tract to the colon. The contractions are created by the muscular wall of the stomach, which consists of inner circular and outer longitudinal smooth muscle.

Stress in all its shapes and sizes, toxins that we feed our body, undigested food particles, pharmaceuticals and pathogens all create gut inflammation, which causes food intolerance and immune-system issues and auto-immunity. So at the heart of your auto-immune issues is most probably a gut malfunction. If you have been struggling with food sensitivities and eliminating those foods and it makes no difference, if you have joint pain and fatigue and the anti-inflammatories are making no difference, if you suffer from skin issues like rosacea or acne and the creams don't work, or if you suffer from weight gain and the diet makes no difference – you probably want to address your gut health now!

Did you know?

The human being is the only animal that has to push faeces uphill against gravity.

What is my microbiome?

The microbiome is a whole inner world that lives within your in-testines and is made up of trillions of tiny microbes that help you extract nutrients from your food, which in turn help balance your mood and your emotions so you can keep a strong clarity and focus on life. By eating food that your gut likes, you will be naturally more productive, more energised, feel brighter and have clearer skin. You can keep your microbiome balanced by eating a mixture of probiotic and prebiotic food.

The relationship between organs in the body is endlessly inter-twined and I think it is important to understand these relationships and where they stem from. Your head says one thing, your heart says another and your gut says something else. Your head says no more biscuits and suddenly there's one in your mouth. There has been a lot of information about the brain and the gut in recent years, and it obviously isn't a new subject as humans have always had both brains and guts, but the enteric nervous system (ENS) was discovered over 150 years ago.

The enteric nervous system is probably the least-known part of the human body and yet it sounds really cool, like something you definitely want to learn more about. In fact, you could say the gut has a mind of its own. The ENS is found in the sheaths of tissue that line the entire gastrointestinal system from the mouth to the anus, roughly measuring about 9 metres (30 feet) and containing more neurons than you would find in the spinal cord. So much is hidden in the gut – from our emotions and feelings to the little that is known about its workings. The ENS sends and receives impulses, records experiences and responds to feelings and emotions. It is full of neurotransmitters and, like the brain, is immediately responsive to stress. This system acts independently as if it had its own body. Dr Michael Gershon, who studies neurogastroenterology, coined the term 'second brain' in 1996.

How to increase the diversity of your microbiome

It sounds strange but you can increase the population of species in the microbiome as well as the diversity of species, as proven by Dr Tim Spector.[3]

If you can, imagine your gut like a flower bed with an array of beautiful roses from all over the world. You would see different co-lours, sizes, shapes of petals, thorns; some would require different soil, water quantities, etc. The point is they are all different. They all need to live together and so you need to learn what each of them needs. Confirmation that you are doing this well would be a positive mood and weight. Signs that you are not being very successful are potentially being overweight, tired and grumpy!

If your rose garden has more roses (good bacteria) than weeds (bad bacteria) then your microbiome is in good shape and will flourish for you. When you test your microbiome with the GI-MAP test I have mentioned earlier (see page 265), you can instantly become in charge of what is going into your body. You can work out what the gut doesn't want – like parasites, pathogenic bacteria, yeast overgrowth and fungal infections – and work out what to repopulate the gut with, such as good bacteria to increase the diversity of the microbiome; digestive enzymes to reinoculate the gut; hydrochloric acid to assist in the breakdown of protein. You might learn that you need to repair the mucosal lining if it has been damaged by food intolerances, parasites or infections. But most importantly you're empowered to rebalance your life and environment so that in future you won't let your defences down and let the bad gut bugs back into you. Creating an environment that the good bugs can hang out in is a mirror of you, your relationships and your boundaries that you have created in life. Having this knowledge allows you not only to take charge of your health by creating a happy gut but you get to make yourself your top priority to create a happier, more comfortable and enjoyable life.

Let's look at how you can grow your gut into a beautiful blossoming flower bed.

Top tips to increase your microbiome diversity

Eat polyphenols: The master antioxidants and the preferred food source for the microbes. Red wine, dark chocolate, dark berries, nuts and seeds.

Get a pet: We all like to be clean and have good hygiene principles but is our obsession with being clean depleting our microbiome? This is where having a pet, especially a dog, could come in handy. Dogs roll around on the grass in mud and bring all those microbes into the house which keep us healthy.

Rewild yourself: A common phrase used in 'microbiome circles', it basically refers to getting back to nature and using the resources of the land – walking, camping, growing crops, farming, foraging and bird watching – which all give us great exposure to germs. De-city yourself for a happy gut!

Eat different foods every week: Humans can really be averse to change. On average I would say most people eat the same breakfast every day and have 2–3 different lunch and dinner options. By having 21 different meals a week think of how many more foods you would eat. The higher the variety of fruits and vegetables, the more strains of microbes you are putting into your body.

Microbiome walk: Have a walk each week to the nearest park, through the forest, into the countryside, but go to a place where you can see foliage, bushes, grass, tracks and trees as far as the horizon and roll around on the land. Leave the phone at home, but leave a note on the kitchen table to let people know where you have gone!

Eat cultured/fermented foods (see list on pages 285-6): Some countries have an advantage over us, like the Koreans with their kimchi, the Germans with their sauerkraut and the Swiss with their dairy and yoghurt produce, but the Japanese[4] win hand over fist with their highly cultured and fermented diet – it's no wonder they live the longest!

Grow your own herbs: This is your first small step to creating your herbal pharmacy on your windowsill, garden, allotment or fields, and this is because the plant world has its own microbiome that we share when we get our hands dirty in the soil. You will also decrease your plastic footprint, increase the variety and flavour of your cooking and start a new hobby. You can even call it herbal meditation!

Play Poohsticks: A childhood game that you play in the microbiome of the country and a favourite of Winnie-the-Pooh! You all choose a stick for its streamline and furiously fast characteristics and throw them into the water over the side of a bridge at the same time, the winner being the person whose stick appears from under the bridge first! This is a favourite on the Somerset Gut Retreat, mixing childhood fun with adult passion and competitiveness.

ENERGIES OF THE GIT

The meridian of the small intestine

The small intestine meridian starts from the little finger of the hand and the outer border of the arm with a zig-zag across the shoulder, neck and up into the face. The small intestine meridian, if out of balance, can affect the intestines and cause intestinal distress, shoulder pain, abdominal pain, earaches, tinnitus, tonsillitis and deafness.

> ### Properties of the small intestine meridian
>
> Force: Yang (male)
> Chakra: Solar plexus – personal power, self-will
> Organ body clock: 1–3pm
> Season: Summer and all hot times
> Colours: Red and blue
> Fragrances: Bitter
> Metaphysical lesson: Inner joy

The meridian of the large intestine

The meridian of the large intestine starts from the index finger and travels along the outer arm to the shoulder, the lateral border of the neck and up to the bottom corner of the nose (outer arms, teeth, sinuses). The large intestine meridian can affect the sinuses, teeth, mucus production in digestion and the sense of smell. If the large intestine meridian is out of balance you can experience abdominal pain, constipation, fever, toothache, diarrhoea and a sore throat.

Properties of the large intestine meridian

Force: Yang (male)

Chakra: Solar plexus – personal power, self-will

Organ body clock: 5–7am

Season: Autumn

Colours: White and yellow

Fragrances: Clove

Metaphysical lesson: Letting go

THE FOUR BODIES OF THE GASTROINTESTINAL SYSTEM

The spiritual body

The large intestine's number one function in the body is to 'let go' – quite literally in a physical sense, to eliminate waste through the movement of peristalsis, but also on a spiritual level, by letting go of the things that don't serve us anymore. This can be people, traits, addictions, food and exercise, or all of the above. Mechanically, the gut lets go of waste after our upper digestive system has taken all the necessary nutrients out of the food we eat. On a spiritual level, the large intestine does the exact same thing. A healthy large intestine energy allows us to let go of patterns of negative thinking, destructive emotions and spiritual blockages that we create which prevent us from being our best. When the function of the large intestine energy is compromised, people have a hard time moving on from difficult situations, or hold very tightly to emotions they know are harming them. Years of constipation issues and not being open with friends and family or letting go can often go hand in hand.

Action: At the Gut Clinic, all clients get a journal to write their thoughts, feelings, desires and plans in. At the beginning or end of the day simply write a few things down to leave more room for new thought, creativity and space. It's just like spring-cleaning your brain!

The emotional body

Knowing how closely the gut and the brain interact, it is easy to understand why you might feel as if you have butterflies in your tummy before a race, or feel nausea before a presentation or interview. This does not mean that your functional gastrointestinal conditions are imagined or are even in your head. Psychology and physical factors combine to cause symptoms of the bowel. The whole gut is influenced by psychological factors that influence the physiology of the gut and create symptoms.

Action: Start your day with a positive affirmation. Look in the mirror and say with strength and conviction and belief, 10 times: 'I let go of the past and I move freely into the present.'

The nutritional body

A vast community of life lives in the dark, oxygen-free zone of our guts, and what you feed this zone will play a large part in how you feel for every second and minute of the day. Scientists say that there are over 100 trillion microbes living in our brains, and it is these microbes that keep the lines of communication open between our heads and our guts and, most importantly, play a very important role in how we feel. If you put in good nutrition you are more likely to feel happy and upbeat, feeding your microbiome for the better; but if you put in food that doesn't rot, you will experience moments, bouts, episodes and even prolonged episodes of the blues because the food will make you feel this way.

Action: Make sure you eat fresh, seasonal, organic fruit and vegetables. Eating foods that decompose means that they have a high life force and will be feeding you high doses of antioxidants, polyphenols, vitamins and minerals. If your tomato can stay in the fridge for over a week with no sign of turning to the dark side, be afraid of the chemicals that have been sprayed on him! If you want to make counting part of your diet, count the chemicals not the calories.

The physical body

In the physical body you may experience the following symptoms, if you're experiencing symptoms with your gut: stiff or tense muscles in the neck as well as headaches. You may also have tight hip flexors.

The main muscle of the hip flexors is a deep muscle called the psoas major, which lies right next to the small intestine. If the psoas muscle is short and tight due to poor posture, poor exercise choices and nutrition, it will enhance visceroptosis. This is when the internal organs drop down into the pelvic basin, creating pelvic floor strain and dysfunction. This muscle can play a role in the gut–brain connection, affecting what is commonly called 'gut feelings'. A tight psoas major muscle may be the cause of your poor motility; it runs from your lumbar spine T12–L4 and inserts/attaches to the lesser trochanter of the femur.

Action: Breathing squats are a great way to fire up the gut and get moving, preferably outside in the morning, but whenever you are feeling sluggish it works, too.

SIGNS THAT YOUR GIT IS UNDER STRESS OR UNHAPPY

Constipation: Inconsistent and infrequent hard-to-pass stools that are dry and can cause the anus to bleed. The cause is tenfold but can stem from straining while having a bowel movement and can result in severe faecel impaction or, at worst, a rectal prolapse.

Diarrhoea: Loose and frequent watery stools which increase the motility of the colon. This condition can be due to a microbial infection, fat absorption issues, nervousness or anxiety.

Inadequate bile secretions: These can lead to a build-up of toxicity in the body and impair fat absorption. Since bile is the agent that lowers toxicity, a deficiency can lead to liver congestion.

Mucorrhoea: Increased cervical discharge lasting 3–4 days, which can be symptomatic of a bacterial overgrowth or infection in the GIT.

Flatulence: It is not uncommon to fart, and we all do it, but there is a difference between the odd puff and chronic smelly farting! Farting is part of the fermentation of small pieces of undigested foods by the bacteria in the small intestines. Fermentation produces gases, which are what cause the smell; these are methane and hydrogen sulphide, which is the rotten-egg smell. Drinking carbonated water, chewing gum and whipped foods all create trapped air and cause us to fart, too.

Small intestinal bacterial overgrowth (SIBO): SIBO is an excessive build-up of bacteria in the SI which can interfere with absorption and digestion. The small intestine is the longest part of the gastrointestinal tract, and although we do see beneficial bacteria in the small intestine, it is mostly found in the colon. Excess amounts can cause severe symptoms of bloating and nausea and nutritional deficiencies as the build-up of bacteria prevents absorption.

Chronic fatigue: Can be a result of all of the above. If you are constipated you are creating toxicity in the body, the liver will become impaired and you will feel tired. If you have diarrhoea you are losing electrolytes, vitamins and minerals, which all give you energy. If you have SIBO or chronic flatulence the energy is being diverted to the area of the gastrointestinal tract where there is an issue, leaving you fatigued. If the root cause is not found you can become chronically fatigued.

Emotions: It is widely accepted that you eat depending on how you feel, and how you feel depends largely on what you have been eating. Eating is one of the most emotional things that we do as *Homo sapiens* – we eat almost more than any other thing that we do. So you need to decide if your food heals or hinders you.

Mood problems: In David Perlmutter's book, *The Grain Brain*[5], he cites scientific papers linking the bacteria in our guts to mental and neurological problems including depression, anxiety and even autism, though he agrees more study is needed to cement the link.

Nutritional eating plan for a healthy gut microbiome

A robust microbiome helps you improve digestion, metabolism, immunity and happiness.

Meals and snacks	Nutrition	Benefits
On waking in the morning	1 pint of filtered water with a squeeze of lemon 10 minutes before food 1 tablespoon of apple cider vinegar Matcha/green tea with lemon	Full of anti-inflammatory and anti-cancer properties. Matcha/green tea is high in antioxidants
First meal of the day	2 soft-boiled eggs with steamed Tenderstem broccoli and sauerkraut (1 tablespoon)	Full of protein, fat and fibre as well as prebiotics
Snack, if desired	Kefir smoothie with coconut yoghurt, berries, ½ avocado, chia seeds and water	Full of probiotics and enzymes – food for better skin and the gut
Second meal of the day	Chicken and vegetable bone broth with a side of kimchi and steamed greens	Full of probiotic foods that will increase the diversity of the microbiome

Snack	Ginger root, turmeric root, lemon and 1 teaspoon of honey with hot water and a bowl of blueberries	Full of digestive and anti-inflammatory properties
Third meal of the day – no food after 7pm	Sweet potato and cauliflower frittata with crushed garlic, red onion and leeks with grilled/baked sea bass	Full of antibacterial and anti-inflammatory properties
Bedtime / activity	Probiotics and a glass of room-temperature water	Increases good bacteria in the gut microbiome

Ulmus rubra, also known as slippery elm, is commonly used for ulceration and mucosal inflammation of the GIT, genitourinary and respiratory tracts.

The mucilage is the part that is used for the mucosal inflammation/ulceration; it comes from the inner bark and is full of polysaccharides, nutrients and vitamins to help soothe and protect the mucous membranes of the GIT.

Fermented foods for the gut

What you put into your gut is so important; if you do not feed it well you may always feel slightly under the weather, have frequent colds and flu and a level of tiredness you just can't shake off. There are foods that the gut does like and foods it doesn't, so for good bowel health you need to know which is which. If the gut is inflamed, some of the foods you think are good for you can cause irritation to the mucosal lining and also cause the sphincters to relax, which is how you can get acid/bile in the wrong places.

Fermented foods are pungent powerhouses of agents that boost the good bacteria in your gut and therefore help with leaky gut, IBS, weight loss, better skin and stronger immunity. The foods listed below can be added into your diet whenever you like. There is no hard-and-fast rule as to when you should have them or how much; they should simply be enjoyed and used when your body feels like it needs a boost. Personally, I might get through a pot of kimchi once a month, kefir and kombucha once a week, and if I am in a shop that sells Laurie's Sauerkraut then I buy every flavour!

We all know that the freshest foods are the best and ideally we want to eat foods that have come straight out of the sea or off the land onto your plate, but fermented food does not fit into this category; in fact it is far removed. Fermented food such as pickled cucumber and cabbage is left to steep in its own sugars and starches until they become bacteria-boosting agents. These are really beneficial in the gut because that is where the immune system lives.

Kombucha: The Chinese call this an immortal health elixir. It has been around for over 2,000 years and has rich health benefits, such as fighting cancer, reducing arthritis and other degenerative diseases. It's full of fizz and a plethora of microorganisms, about 4–7 different strains, which build a strong gut.

Sauerkraut: Studies show that sauerkraut is not only meant to keep your German sausages company but also reduces depression and anxiety, and that's because of the connection between brain and gut.

Pickles: These are the safe bet of fermented foods and are accepted and recognised as such. They are also full of probiotics. They may be found in a jar at the back of your local bar, might accompany your miso soup in a pot, or be served in your burger.

Miso: This is a paste made from fermented soya beans. Miso is full of potassium which helps to offset the effects of sodium in your diet.

Miso is a great way to start a meal and prepare your digestive system for food.

Tempeh: Similar to miso, tempeh starts as a fermented soya bean and is a complete protein. It will never be a substitute for meat, but nutritionally it does contain all the required amino acids. Add tamari sauce to tempeh to give it extra flavour.

Kimchi: Spicy cabbage doesn't sound inviting but even the thought of this will get your gastric juices flowing. Not only will kimchi heal and repair your gut it will make you look 10 years younger. Remember: if it's good for your gut it's good for your skin.

Kefir: Is a fermented milk drink that can be made from cow's, goat's or sheep's milk to which kefir grains are added. These are not grains as you or I know them but rather cultures of yeast and lactic acid bacteria. Kefir is a powerful probiotic.

DEPRESSION, THE MISSING LINK

In a 2015 study by Dr Bercik and his team at McMaster University, Canada[6], it was discovered that germ-free mice (mice with no gut bacteria) when compared with normal mice displayed anxiety-ridden behaviours. This shows how the role of microbiomes plays an important part in behaviour. The study looked at how a stressful situation in life – in the case of the mice, being separated from their mothers – and how the emotions of depression played a significant part in later life. Abnormal levels of cortisol, the stress hormone, were found, as well as the release of the neurotransmitter acetylcholine, which causes an impaired gut lining. When the scientists transferred gut bacteria from normal mice to the germ-free mice, within weeks the behaviours of anxiety and depression disappeared. What was interesting was the discovery that if the bacteria from stressed mice was transferred into non-stressed, germ-free mice, no abnormalities were observed. As Dr Bercik concluded, 'This suggests that . . . both host and microbial factors are required for the development of anxiety and depression-like behaviour.'

When the gut is imbalanced you may present with the following symptoms: procrastination, teeth grinding, incompletion of tasks, changes in addictive behaviours, taking up new addictive behaviours, an increased desire to be withdrawn or away from the company of others. The best way to avoid these symptoms and keep your gut healthy and happy is to take a gastrointestinal test every year that includes GI markers that let you see if your body is trending in or out of health.

PATHOLOGIES OF THE GUT

Blastocystis hominis

Blastocystis hominis is found in humans all over the world; however, most commonly it is found in males and in immune-compromised people. The cysts of B. hominis are 6–40µm in size and gain entry via the mouth from faeces. The cysts then infect the epithelial cells of the digestive tract and multiply asexually. Blasto can remain in the intestine for weeks, months or years.

Blastocystis hominis was once thought to be harmless and a yeast at that, but it is in fact a parasite, a microscopic single-celled organism (protozoan). Protozoans usually inhabit your gastrointestinal tract and are thought to be harmless and even helpful, but others can and do cause symptoms similar to that of IBS. Blasto is found in 30 per cent of people who suffer from IBS and can be asymptomatic, meaning that you do not necessarily have symptoms. You can be fit and healthy and have Blasto, or you can be unhealthy and immune-compromised with it. In children, common signs would be irritability and over-activeness.

Like anything in life, if you create an environment that is attractive you will find it hard to get rid of visitors. The key is to create an environment, a terrain in your gut, that no unwanted or unsavoury characters want to hang around in. If you don't provide any drinks or nibbles for your guests at a party they probably won't stay very long, and it's the same in your gut. If you continue to feed yourself foods high in refined sugar and starch you will be providing a constant supply of food for the bugs.

A parasite is an organism that feeds off another organism, called a host. The major groups of parasites include protozoans (organisms having only one cell) and parasitic worms (helminths) and each of these parasites can infect the digestive tract, and sometimes two or more can cause infection at the same time. Intestinal parasites populate the gastrointestinal tract in humans and other animals. They can live throughout the body, but most prefer to inhabit the intestinal wall. Means of exposure include ingestion of undercooked meat, drinking infected water and skin absorption. There are many treatments available for intestinal parasites but the vitality of the person and the environment of their gut are the two most important things to look at before designing a plan of attack.

What *Blastocystis hominis* infections/parasites might look or feel like

All these symptoms are not exclusive to *Blastocystis hominis*, so clinical testing would be needed to confirm the diagnosis, as is true of all pathologies as they share many signs and symptoms.

Swelling of facial features and of the body: If certain parasites invade the intestinal tract they can release toxins into the body – this can lead to an increase of the eosinophils levels in your blood, which can be the reason behind sores, lesions, ulcers and swelling on the body and face.

Teeth grinding: There may be many reasons why you grind your teeth. One plausible cause can be intestinal parasites.

Anal itching: This is another sign of a parasite infection and particularly of pinworms – *E. vermicularis*. At night the female pinworms migrate towards the anus, where they lay their eggs. Both the migrating female pinworms as well as the clumps of eggs are irritating and cause itching, crawling sensations or even acute pain. Inside the body, the eggs hatch in the small intestine and take one to two months to mature. Adult pinworms then travel to the large intestine (colon) to mate. At night, typically when their human hosts are asleep, pregnant female pinworms leave the anus to deposit their eggs in the perianal area.

Chronic fatigue: If you are struggling with fatigue and no matter what you try it doesn't improve, you might have a parasite. Parasites can deplete your energy because they feed off your food supply, making you feel weak and tired. This can lead to absorption issues, i.e. an inability to assimilate and absorb all the nutrients and vitamins from your food. Over time the fatigue can lead to mental and physical exhaustion and also affect your emotional status, especially if you are actively trying to resolve your tiredness by your own means. So if you're experiencing this, make sure you seek help.

Change in appetite and weight loss: We often joke that we could do with a worm infection as a quick solution to weight loss! Weight loss is often a symptom of a worm infection but also a change in appetite can be due to the presence of a parasite. So keep a check on your weight.

Mood disorders: The gut is, as we have seen, the emotional centre of the body and so when the gut starts to get infected and its protective measures become impaired our mood can dramatically change, too. One of the reasons this happens is because living in the GIT is one of our neurotransmitters called serotonin, which is our happy hormone, and these levels can deplete.[6] Neurons also line the gut and are responsible for a healthy enteric nervous system. New research is constantly emerging that inflammation in the gut can lead to inflammation in the brain.

Iron-deficiency anaemia: Parasites steal vitamins, including iron, from the food the person eats, leading to an iron deficiency. Infections by intestinal roundworms or pinworms can lead to iron deficiency in the body and ultimately cause anaemia.

Rectal prolapse: A prolapse occurs when the last part of the wall of the colon collapses just before the anus and starts to protrude through the anus. You can have a part or whole rectal prolapse.

Insomnia: Any sleep issues, including not being able to get to sleep or stay asleep.

Case study

Bloody *Blasto!*

Kevin called me from Australia after he had seen some of the work and results I had been getting with clients at the Gut Clinic in London. He had tested positively for *Blastocystis hominis* over the last five years by three different hospitals and was getting a bit fed up.

I needed him to do one more test so I could see the severity of the infection and what else had invited themselves to this party in his gut. There is never just one bug partying alone!

Kevin had had malaria when he was nine years old, glandular

fever when he was 16 and various surgeries between the ages of 16 and 19 for shoulder stabilisations. He also had his appendix removed when he was 17. It was at the age of 17 that he noticed his health was starting to suffer, and he made particular reference to his glands flaring up. He was someone who would have been a contender for a parasite infection based just on his international travel: Hong Kong was home and he travelled extensively through South-east Asia during his school years. He had settled in New Mexico before moving to the Middle East and then Australia, and had travelled to the majority of countries in Europe and Africa, too. An envious travel schedule!

Here is his story and health history in his words.

Stomach issues: I have suffered from severe stomach pain, bloating, cramps and occasional bleeding sporadically between 2000 and 2015 (at times okay, at other times I've had terrible issues). I have experienced common bouts of diarrhoea, even when there were no other symptoms. I tried several other solutions, from using over-the-counter pharmacy drugs (Gaviscon) to natural solutions like peppermint oil and tea, but nothing had any impact. I saw several gastro experts in 2012, who wanted to perform a colonoscopy and suggested that surgery was probably needed based on my symptoms.

I have lived with low-level or flaring symptoms for over 15 years, and while the pain and discomfort were highly frustrating, it was often the sense of not knowing what was wrong that caused the most anxiety for me. The symptoms would flare frequently and could be very severe at times; the combination of the duration of the symptoms and the sporadic pain was very tough to cope with and I really didn't know what to do. I contacted GPs, natural remedy specialists, gastroenterologists, all of whom failed to diagnose me with anything concrete. I tried several diet changes including going gluten- and lactose-free, neither of which cleared the symptoms. I was beginning to think this was something I would just have to live with for the rest of my life.

Luckily, I came across some blog posts by Hannah about her work on the gut and the role of parasites, which was backed up by her work with Dr Omar Amin. I contacted Hannah early in 2015, and after a few quick tests, Hannah tested for and found severe *Blastocystis hominis*. At first it was a relief to have a diagnosis, even better was that Hannah had a plan and told me she knew how to kill it (but it could be a bitch to kill). I started immediately on the protocol for gut/immune support that she wrote for me, along with a diet and lifestyle plan. Even though I ended up travelling a lot during this treatment (to Indonesia of all places, parasite heaven), and my work stress levels were high, I stuck to the treatment and at my next round of tests, only five months later, Hannah confirmed my symptoms had been cleared. I'm ecstatic at the fact I don't have to deal with this for life, and that the treatment was so pain- (and surgery-) free! I can't thank Hannah enough for her help and support, and mostly her confidence that this could be cured. It's opened my eyes up to thinking about my health in so many new ways. Thanks, Hannah!

Lifestyle plan for the prevention of parasites

Prevention	How / why
Always wash your hands after going to the toilet, dealing with babies and before you cook or prepare food	Use warm water and soap; I like the grapefruit handwash by Bentley Organic

Always wash vegetables and fruits	With warm water and a scrubbing brush
Drink bottled water while in developing countries	To prevent contamination
Make sure your bins have lids on and are thrown out bi-weekly	As infection can be airborne and cultivated in warm environments
Always keep your toothbrush in a cupboard	Spores can be infectious
Pets with ill health	Will easily pick up infection and spread to you when they lick you
Sex	Always take protection
Always close the toilet seat	As spores can be infectious

How can I tell if I have a worm?

You may very well be itching your bum, especially at night, if you have a worm. Pinworm (*Enterobius vermicularis*) is one of the most common infections in humans. They are white worms less than a centimetre (½ inch) long which live in the large intestine of adults and children. The worms reproduce sexually and can produce up to 10,000 fertilised eggs. At night the pregnant female migrates out of the anus and onto the skin of the buttocks, where she expels all of her eggs and then dies. The majority of the eggs stay on the skin, but some will fall onto the bed linen and some will go airborne, and these eggs can mature within six hours of being laid. Are you itching?!

As you sleep you start to itch and the eggs get trapped under the fingernails, so if you do not wash your hands and you then eat with your hands you will simply reinfect yourself as you swallow the pinworms. The life cycle lasts 4–6 weeks.

Other symptoms of a worm infection include nausea, weakness, abdominal pain, fatigue, diarrhoea and vitamin and mineral deficiencies. However, as with many illnesses, the infection can be asymptomatic. One way to be sure would be either testing in a laboratory or by looking for segments of the worms that pass in your stools. If the infection is large, it can sometimes block the intestines. With pork tapeworm larvae, once they move out of the intestines they can migrate to other parts of the body.

IBS: Irritable bowel syndrome

A common, long-term condition which can be recognised by symptoms of abdominal pain and cramping relieved by passing stools, diarrhoea, constipation (sometimes both), bloating, flatulence, urgency, incomplete emptying of bowels and mucus in the stools. It can be caused by an increased sensitivity of the gut, an ulceration of the gut and problems digesting food, a previous allergy or GIT infection as well as an emotional trauma or life event.

There are generally two categories of IBS you will fall into: IBS – constipation; or IBS – diarrhoea.

What IBS might look or feel like to you

Abdominal pain: Any of the following symptoms can come under abdominal pain, such as bloating, flatulence and cramping relieved by passing stools.

Urgency: Urgency for the bathroom is a common sign of IBS. Here the lining of the digestive system is irritated, caused by food intolerance, lactose intolerance, infection or constipation (straining over time leads to weak and slack muscles).

Chronic fatigue: Due to the fact that you may not be efficiently absorbing your nutrients in the digestive tract and so your food is not nourishing you and giving you energy.

Bloating/swelling of the stomach: This can happen immediately as you eat food, during a meal or after a meal. You may look more bloated in the evening, too – both are indications of problems in the digestive tract.

Allopathic treatment for IBS

Omeprazole is a proton pump inhibitor (PPI) and one of the top 10 most widely used drugs in the world that can decrease levels of beneficial bacteria in the gut, causing infection, and has now been found to have a worse effect on the gut than previously thought. The problem is that many drugs are not taken appropriately and often additional advice is not given with the drug, so it offers the solution when in fact it can end up exacerbating a person's health. In a study by Floris Imhann in 2015 on the effect of PPIs on the microbiome, he found that there was a significant increase in pathogenic bacteria and a reduction in good bacteria species in the gut bacteria of clients who had been prescribed these drugs.[8]

Naturopathic plan for IBS/C (constipation)

If you experience constipation with your IBS, follow these suggestions:

- Increase your fluid intake and avoid caffeine, due to its diuretic action.
- Create a regular and consistent eating time to encourage regular elimination.
- If the following are lacking in your diet, make sure to include whole grains, steamed vegetables, fruits and legumes and rice bran, as all can increase stool mass. Natural laxatives can work for some people and you would need to trial-and-error these, such as prunes, figs, apricots and rhubarb.
- Supplements for laxative effect: magnesium citrate and vitamin C, B5, saffron and ginger.
- Increase your bile flow: inositol, choline and methionine, omega 3s (EPA/DHA).
- Take probiotics – these can help improve motility through the bowel.

Naturopathic plan for IBS/D (diarrhoea)

If you experience diarrhoea with your IBS, follow these suggestions. If you have chronic diarrhoea you can also be at risk of associated malabsorption of essential nutrients and therefore supplementation should be considered, including magnesium, iron, potassium, sodium, zinc, vitamins A, B12 and C, and copper.

- Increase your fibre intake and perhaps consider taking psyllium husk, a soluble fibre providing a bulk-forming laxative.
- Eat fruits and vegetables in abundance rather than legumes and cereal grains.
- Consider taking a food allergy (IgE) or intolerance (IgG) test.

The good news with IBS is that it is all so manageable, preventable and reversible. So if you have been told you have it, you now know what to do to make the positive changes.

Case study

What your doctor won't tell you

An urgency for a bowel movement with little warning not only became an inconvenient symptom but also an embarrassing one for Lucy, who I met on the TV series *Don't Tell the Doctor*. In fact, it had got so bad that recently Lucy had had an 'accident' at a restaurant with friends and her new boyfriend! She had been suffering from IBS for six years when I was asked to see if I could make some changes to her diet and lifestyle in order for her to reduce stress, lose weight and ultimately get out of pain. She was suffering with these painful flare-ups of constipation, extreme diarrhoea and constant bloating, which was beginning to affect her work and social life. She would often have to cancel plans as the constant need for the bathroom was becoming unbearable and the bloating was affecting her confidence – she looked pregnant and her skin was getting her down.

It struck me that she could definitely make some changes to her diet and lifestyle, which alone would go a long way to helping her feel fitter, lighter and more confident. I suspected a yeast overgrowth and so, as is protocol at the Gut Clinic, sent off a stool sample for an Invivo GI-MAP test for yeast, bacteria, parasites and inflammation.

I saw Lucy a month later and, against the odds of having a cold and a virus over Christmas, she had lost 2.2kg – nearly 5 pounds – and the bloated look had gone, she said, except when the cheeky panini crept in! Well, this is real life, after all. I asked her how she was feeling about her skin and she said that she no longer felt like a monster when she took her make-up off. (Gut issues do not confine themselves to the gut; they spread far and wide and the skin takes on this emotional aftermath.)

This was music to my ears. Lucy was a cheery person but I felt that the cheeriness had been a cover for actually feeling sad inside. She certainly was feeling happy now. Before there had been takeaways and ready meals every night, but now she was in the kitchen with her partner cooking from scratch! Cooking is one of the best skills you can acquire; if you can cook you can feed yourself, make yourself strong, be in charge of your happiness, how you feel, and you also get to spend time with either yourself or your partner. As a couple they connected more; they were taking walks in the country each week and at the weekend, as well as taking a yoga class and using the stairs at work.

When the tests came back from the laboratory a yeast overgrowth was found and everything she had been experiencing, the bloating, the tiredness, the skin outbreaks, the foggy thinking and bloating, started to fall into place. I made changes to her diet to eliminate some of the high-sugar options she was going for but made sure that this was a process rather than a cold-turkey approach. Often if you embark on an elimination diet when you have previously been living in the biscuit tin you will inevitably set yourself up for failure. So I made sure that I kept some of her creature comforts, for a little while until we could replace them with things she enjoyed even more that didn't carry the same outcomes.

Leaky gut syndrome: increased intestinal permeability

Leaky gut affects the whole body, it is not just confined to the gut. It could actually be the cause of some other health problems you may be experiencing. Chronic fatigue, food allergies, joint pain, auto-immune disease and weight gain can all be because of leaky gut.

Imagine going fishing with a huge net; the river is swimming with fish all ready to be caught and to feed beautiful you, except your net has been damaged and now has a large hole in it, allowing dead fish, pond weed and the bugs to get through. Your gut lining works just like the fishing net; it is a barrier that keeps out all the bigger particles that can damage your system. The key is not to eat foods that cause inflammation to this lining.

Leaky gut syndrome is a term not liked by the medical profession but it sums up the problem with no confusion: the gut is leaking!

When the gut lining is damaged, proteins such as gluten, undigested food particles and pathogenic bacteria can pass through into the bloodstream. The immune system can also take a hit as toxic waste can leak from the inside of your intestinal wall, causing an immune reaction.

It starts when the intestinal wall of the gut is compromised and creates inflammation-causing malabsorption of certain nutrients such as B12, magnesium and iron. The body responds by creating an immune response as a way of saying 'help me!', but in the meantime

GI issues have started and you may also be struggling with many food intolerances as your body is not efficiently breaking down the food for absorption. Food intolerances are created when you lack the specific enzyme to break down the protein; for example, if you bloat when you drink milk you are probably insufficient in the enzyme lactose.

What leaky gut might look or feel like to you
Nutritional deficiencies: The main ones will be B12, zinc and digestive enzymes. You may start to notice that your hair is getting drier, as is your skin.

Food intolerances: Multiple food sensitivities are a red flag for leaky gut. If you eat a food and you get a reaction – whether you bloat, go red, get a rash or your breathing rate increases – you need to address the issue. This is a very clear sign that your body does not like the food and has created an immune response to it, and if left untreated or undiagnosed it will escalate into a more serious gut malfunction.

How to test for leaky gut
Zonulin: This is considered a biomarker of increased intestinal hyperpermeability (leaky gut), and elevated levels have been found in coeliac disease. Leaky gut is a condition that can occur when the gut lining becomes abnormally permeable – it's like someone not shutting the doors to a club and letting all the riff-raff in. Toxins, unwanted food particles and other harmful substances that should not have been given entry get to cross over into the bloodstream because of the gaps that start to develop between the intestines and the bloodstream.

How to heal your leaky gut
A lot of people come to see me because they have one or more digestive issues that they no longer want to put up with. They may find

that they can no longer lose weight like they used to or that they have stopped being able to digest heavy fats and proteins as they once did. They may also come because they are finding more and more foods are contributing to their symptoms, and so cooking, eating and eating out are becoming less pleasurable and – in fact – stressful. Often clients just want to be told what to eat, but the more I help people with digestive issues, the more the recovery seems to lie in the way people live their lives, conduct their relationships and value themselves, rather than being about the actual food. The modern-day lifestyle, the pressure and the stress of finding your own place in the world has put a considerable amount of stress on our digestive tracts, leaving us in a very emotional and vulnerable place of health.

So before you do anything else, look at the list below and ask yourself how often do you do any or all of the strategies to create the right environment for your gut, and to bring calm and serenity to your life.

- Walking in nature: a park, forest, woodland, the countryside.
- Being by yourself each day with no electronics or music, TV or entertainment.
- Allowing time each day for meditation.
- Making a pot of tea with fresh ingredients – mint and lemon or turmeric and honey.
- Write down all your worries, thoughts and wishes in a journal every night.
- Journalling every day, allowing thoughts to turn into words, which turn into deeds.
- Doing hobbies such as putting together puzzles, knitting or learning an instrument, to keep the mind active and the body moving without being in a stressful environment.
- Ignoring distractions while eating: being away from technology, books or other activities.
- Savouring food by taking in the smell, the flavour and the texture before the first bite.

Perhaps you already do some of these things, but if you are not doing any of these it might be time to start putting one or more of them into practice and build up from there.

Yeast overgrowth

Yeast, fungi and parasites are ubiquitous in nature: they are everywhere, you cannot possibly be free of parasites or fungi completely. If you did manage somehow to do this you would probably have worse health than with them. The key is to create a balanced relationship with them. A strong immune system can deal with these extra organisms but when the immune system drops and the sugar intake goes up, an infection can often set in, which is when you may have a problem.

Yeast overgrowths are common these days and even more common among vegetarians and vegans. You may be familiar with some of the symptoms: a white tongue, itching, fungus in the toes, vaginal discharge, mucus around ovulation time for females and penile yeast infection.

Predisposing factors for a yeast overgrowth are high-sugar and starch diets, a compromised immune system, nutrient deficiency, impaired liver function and altered bowel states. By reducing the amount of sugar and starch in your diet you can starve the overgrowth, preventing proliferation. A yeast overgrowth can cause toxicity and these toxins can travel to virtually all tissues and areas of the body. Candida is a yeast that produces fungal mycotoxins, a group of naturally occurring chemicals produced by certain moulds that we eat, such as cereals, nuts, spices, dried fruits, apple juice and coffee. These foods are often stored or cultivated under warm and humid conditions, which allows the mould to grow.

THE RITUAL OF EATING: A LOST PASTIME

One of my main pieces of advice to my clients is to use the dinner table as a place to sit with friends and/or family and give thanks or grace for the food that is about to be eaten, and to celebrate life and the people who are sitting with you. Many of my clients eat around their computers, slumped over their keyboards, not even noticing the food they're consuming or how quickly they're doing it – yet it is lifestyle habits like this that contribute to digestive disorders and issues.

People often ask me what the best advice is for digestion, and this is what I tell them.

Digestion rules:

- Sit down at a table to eat, without your phone, the TV, your laptop, or Netflix. Leave work and stress in your laptop, never eat with it open.
- Drink water before you eat and sip to cleanse the palate (don't gulp it).
- Always have a green leafy steamed vegetable on your plate.
- Chew your food to liquid – take your time, enjoy and savour the food, appreciate the flavours and textures and be present when you are having dinner. If you are a fast eater, be the last to finish.

Let the cleansing begin

First of all you have to know what you are cleansing from, which is why clinical testing is a good place to start. Of course, you can do the gut cleanse without knowing what exactly is going on in your gut, but I like to know to what degree you need to use supplements, herbal remedies, lifestyle changes, and to fine-tune the nutritional/diet requirements rather than guessing. The gut can play host to bacteria, excessive yeast, fungi overgrowths and even parasites. Once the invaders have leached over into the bloodstream they will start to deplete your energy, overwork your immune system and create inflammation by attaching themselves to the intestinal walls. So if you can't remember the last time you felt on top of the world I would advise you to do some clinical testing. The GI-MAP test from Invivo Clinical or PCI Europe is a perfect way to start the year. Just like you take your car in for an MOT, we should really be doing the same service on our bodies.

Remember not to compare yourself to others as you start to clean up your diet. You are changing the environment of your gut, and what works for one may not work for another. All cleanses will go through some trial and error until you can see what is working and what is not working. It is also important to feel that your vitality is high before embarking on a fungal/parasite cleanse so that you have the energy to get rid of the unwanted guests!

Step 1: remove what your gut and life do not want

The remove phase focuses on removing fungi, pathogenic bacteria, parasites, viruses, allergens and toxins from the GIT. Remember, it is not about removing everything at once; it's about making a change in the right direction, and this is the first step.

Remove the following from your kitchen/cupboards/life:

- Microwaves.
- Stressful situations.
- Gluten grains: couscous, barley, spelt, kamut, farro, durum, bulgur, rye, triticale, semolina.
- Alcohol; if you can't give it up altogether, make sure your beer and wine is organic and gluten-free, your spirits are clear and you have more days without than with.
- Caffeine; if you can't give this up, make sure the coffee you buy is organic and ground, never instant.
- Over-exercising.
- Bad energy – toxic people and environments.
- Late nights and early mornings – swap these for early nights and early mornings.
- Pollution, where possible.
- Eating out at restaurants such as fast-food places and getting takeaways.
- Cow's dairy – all products.

By testing you can remove the problem and start getting on with repairing and rebalancing your gut and your life. On testing you may find one or all of the issues below:

- Food intolerances
- Pathogenic bacteria
- Fungi
- Parasites

Step 2: replace what is missing in your kitchen/cupboards/life

The replace phase is the part that focuses on replenishing what is lacking in the body, to aid efficient digestion. Mainly that will look like replacing enzymes or acid, two of the substances that allow food to be broken down into smaller particles for absorption. Digestive enzymes can be broken down into three categories:

- Protease, responsible for breaking down protein.
- Lipase, responsible for breaking down fat.
- Amylase, responsible for breaking down carbohydrates.

These enzymes are usually secreted by the pancreas and when they are in short supply digestive symptoms, such as bloating, undigested food in stools or constipation, may arise.

Having a pantry full of the essentials is key to building good practices around preparing and making food. I've made a list of all the essentials I have in my pantry at home and I would also suggest that for your fresh produce you support your nearest local fresh-food places, such as a fishmonger, butcher and greengrocer.

Make sure you have these essentials:

- Sea salt and ground black pepper.
- A selection of garden herbs and spices and fresh herbs, growing on the windowsill or dried.
- Coconut oil, olive oil, ghee.
- Apple cider vinegar, tamari sauce, chutneys, ginger and turmeric root (fresh and dried).

- Brown rice, basmati rice, lentils, quinoa, pulses, legumes, beans.
- Tins/jars of tomatoes, tomato puree, tuna, sardines, coconut milk.
- Vegetables and fruits – in small amounts, as ideally you want to buy these daily.
- Keep garden peas, mixed vegetables, soups and bone broths (home-cooked in batches (see page 81) and frozen in portions) in your freezer.

Replace the contents of your kitchen and cupboards with:

- Bitter foods: Swedish bitters, watercress, rocket and dandelion. All these foods stimulate the production of enzymes and bile flow to aid digestion.
- Apple cider vinegar: Take 1 tablespoon 10 minutes before meals, neat or in 50ml (2fl oz) of water.
- Zinc and B6; both are needed for the production of pancreatic enzymes and hydrochloric acid, the acid that lives in your stomach and is responsible for protein breakdown, among other things.
- B12 and intrinsic factor.

Step 3: replenish with prebiotics and probiotics

Prebiotics and probiotics work synergistically together, and for best results can be taken together. They are often described as friendly, beneficial or healthy, and that is exactly what they are – they are the safest way to keep a healthy intestinal ecosystem balanced. Other ways to support the gut are eating a varied diet of fresh seasonal fruits, vegetables and wholefoods.

Replenish your gut with these:

- *Lactobacillus*
- *Lactobacillus reuteri*
- *Bifidobacterium infantis*
- *Saccharomyces boulardii*
- Prebiotics

Then replenish your kitchen cupboards with fermented foods – see the list of recommended foods on pages 285–6 – as well as supplements such as probiotics, which must be taken regularly for change to be seen and for them to promote health. Keep your probiotics in the fridge, as bacteria are delicate. This ensures a longer life of the product and better efficiency, too.

- Olives
- Raw vinegars
- Ginger and root beer
- Traditional sourdough breads
- Wheatgrass juice
- Natural yoghurt
- Black tea and oolong tea
- Pickles

Foods and herbs that are rich in polyphenols also increase the beneficial bacteria in the gut. Polyphenols give colour to the food, such as green tea, red wine, apples, onions, chocolate and black tea.

Top tip: If you start bloating when taking a probiotic, persevere. When disease-producing fungi or bacteria die, they release chemicals that can cause bloating to worsen – this as known as a die-off reaction. If this happens, reduce your intake and gradually build up your dose.

Step 4: repair the wall of the gut

This is the phase that is often forgotten about. We get rid of what we don't want or what is causing us a problem, and when that's done we can be mistaken for thinking that is the end of the job. Do not make this mistake!

If you always do what you have always done, you will always get what you have always got - bugs!

If you do not change the environment it is only a matter of time before a similar issue rears its ugly head and you start getting gut pain again. The repair phase is of paramount importance.

So, repair your kitchen and cupboards with some of the following supplements:

- Antioxidants: fill up on fresh fruit and vegetables, especially the brightly coloured ones.
- Zinc: you can leave zinc tablets by your bedside table for best absorption, or you can get it naturally from proteins, leafy greens, brown rice and nuts.
- L-glutamine: you can use this as a powder and add it to your smoothie or cold-pressed cabbages!
- N-acetylcysteine: a potent antioxidant to support the liver throughout the cleanse. Taking a liver support is important to help clear the excess toxins throughout a cleanse. Must be taken as a supplement.

Step 5: restore and regenerate

Laugh, live and love above all else.

Reduce the things that make you sympathetic dominant (stress) and increase the things that make you parasympathetic dominant (the list below).

Look after beautiful you by doing the following:

- Make time for me-time – do something you enjoy every day.
- Soak in magnesium salt baths with lavender drops and listen to classical music.
- Do hobbies/activities that make you happy.
- Take walks in the countryside or around your local park or nature reserve.
- Meet up with friends who make you happy and give you energy.
- Write a journal at the beginning or end of each day, jotting down your thoughts and feelings.

● Detox your house: throw away objects and clothes that you have not used for six months.

The gut is an emotional little friend who needs constant looking after. If you bombard the gut with poor food choices and poor-quality food you may have to start looking after your gut more often than not. Don't wait for something to go wrong as it may be too late – keep up the maintenance on your body just like you do on your car!

THE GORGEOUS GUT CLEANSE

Do I qualify for a gut cleanse?

We all overeat from time to time, or all the time – for some of us food is on our minds constantly and a large amount of our social lives revolves around food. We overeat for many reasons: because we are bored; unsatisfied with the food we have eaten; are harbouring a bug or yeast infection; have become addicted to sugar in its various guises; or perhaps because we are overstressed or simply depressed.

The gorgeous gut cleanse has been designed to give your digestive system a well-deserved rest – a bit of a holiday from the overtime it does on a regular basis. You might like to try it if you have overeaten, or simply had a lot of celebrations over the weekend and want to feel refreshed by the end of Monday, or you may want to do it for longer.

If you have any outstanding medical conditions, do make sure you consult with a medical/health professional first.

The rules of the gorgeous gut cleanse

You can cleanse for one to four days, the length of time is up to you.

What you eat on a cleanse day

Food intake / day	Recommended time of day	Ingredients and method	Quantity / amount	Lifestyle / sleep / extras
Organic bone broth (see page 81)	Breakfast and dinner	Chicken, beef, fish, mushroom, vegetable Simmer the bones for over 10 hours	2 x 500ml (18fl oz) per day	Aim to be in bed for 10pm and wake at 6am
Cold-pressed juice	Breakfast and mid-afternoon	½ garlic clove, ½ lemon, 2 x celery sticks, 200g (7oz) spinach, 1 apple, ½ broccoli head – flowers and stalk, 1 cucumber Chop into small pieces as required to put through the cold-press juicer	2 x 330ml (11fl oz)	Stretching/ meditation/ yoga/tai-chi/ mobilisations on waking
Apple	Mid-morning and before or after dinner	Organic, seasonal and locally grown if possible	x 2	Magnesium salt bath or lavender bath at night
Herbal tea: fresh root tea	Throughout the day as desired	Fresh tea options: Ginger root Fresh lemon Green, white or black tea Chamomile or lavender flowers Add hot water in a teapot and leave to steep for 4 minutes	As many as you want	Weigh, measure (waist – around the belly button, hips and thighs), take photos of yourself (front and back and face) on the first day and last day

Water	Throughout the day and ideally the majority before 5pm	Filtered	2 litres (3½ pints) at least	Dark chocolate, 70% cocoa solids, 2 squares per day
Cold-pressed anti-ageing and anti-inflammatory juice	Throughout the day as desired	Turmeric and ginger root (1 thumbnail), 1 x unwaxed lemon and rind, water and 1 dessertspoon raw honey, diluted with filtered water	1 litre (1¾ pints) of filtered water	100g (3½ oz) berries – blueberries, raspberries, strawberries or cranberries

What can I eat if my cravings/willpower get the better of me?

- Dark chocolate 70 per cent cocoa solids – maximum 2 squares.
- White fish, grilled or poached – 100g (3½ oz).
- Steamed green vegetables – 200g (7 oz).
- Berries such as blueberries, raspberries, strawberries or cranberries – 100g (3½ oz).

The idea of this one to four-day cleanse is to show you how much better you can feel and your stomach can look and feel in a short space of time. This will help you to start to make some of the things you have learnt during the cleanse second nature in your life, and more regular features of your diet.

What will improve over the four days?

Bloating, bowel movement, foggy thinking, sleep, skin, mood, sugar cravings.

If you eliminate 'snow white' (white flour, white refined sugar, milk, potatoes, dairy products – which of course includes bread, cakes and biscuits of all types and all sugars that end in 'ose') you can stop feeling like the seven dwarfs: grumpy, sleepy, dopey, moody, farty, gassy and bloaty!

TOP 10 TIPS FOR A HEALTHY GASTROINTESTINAL TRACT

1. **Create the cephalic response:** This occurs even before food enters the stomach. The cerebral cortex (the appetite centre) of the brain signals the cephalic phase of gastric secretion in your gut and is stimulated by sight, smell and the thought of food. It reacts by sending a message to the medulla oblongata via the hypothalamus, which then triggers the gastric juices in the stomach wall by alerting the parasympathetic nervous system (PNS) via the vagus nerve, readying them for the arrival of food.

2. **Drink water before you eat:** Drinking water while you eat only dilutes your digestive enzymes, but drinking before a meal stimulates the gastric juices and helps you break down your food. Sipping water in between mouthfuls is fine as a palate cleanser.

3. **Eat protein upon waking:** Starting your day with protein has all-round benefits that satisfy your satiety hormones and regulate your digestive hormones. The protein can come from an animal or a fish source, beans, legumes, dairy or eggs or a protein powder.

4. **Eat small meals:** Your stomach is where all your food gets delivered after you have swallowed it. Your stomach is only small, so it prefers little meals for optimal digestion. If you take your time and chew slowly you will also eat less, and in a world where we are all guilty of overeating, a spot of portion control won't go amiss.

5. **Take a probiotic at night:** We need probiotics because whichever way you look at it, our food is not as pure as it once was, and, however diligent you are at eating organic, seasonal, grass-fed and local food, we still need to redress the balance of gut bacteria as it depletes with modern-day stress. Having a high level of good microbes in the gut keeps your immune system strong, your weight balanced and your inflammation down. Take at night for best reinoculation of the gut, when digestion has finished and repair is about to take place. For this reason it is advised not to eat after 8pm in the evening.

6. **Use fresh herbs and spices:** Herbs and spices can turn something

bland in taste into something wonderful. Grow fresh herbs in your garden and save money or have dried herbs and spices in the pantry. In particular with regard to a healthy gut, ginger will help gastrointestinal distress, fennel will calm indigestion, as well as help with constipation and flatulence, and cumin will help calm bloating and gas.

7. **Juice cabbages:** Without a doubt one of the most medicinal vegetables around. Cabbages are a rich source of phytochemicals that have potent anti-cancer properties. Cabbage juice works wonders for gastric ulcers, diverticulosis and for healing digestive problems in general as it contains sulforaphane, which kills off the bacteria-causing peptic ulcers and helps repair the GIT from gastric reflux.

8. **Optimise your elimination:** Your beautiful body should pass 30 centimetres (12 inches) of faeces a day, which could be all at once in the morning, or twice or three times a day. Optimal elimination is about 1–2 hours after your three main meals, but we are all different. However common it is for people not to have a bowel movement every day, it is not normal and should be addressed immediately. Your bowel health is one of the greatest, easiest indicators of your overall health and guess what – you are in charge, so start having a peek!

9. **Fast once in a while:** Give your digestive system a rest, a day off for good behaviour. Sometimes we are not hungry, sometimes we feel like skipping dinner or lunch, and this is okay. Start listening to your body and feel or hear what it is asking you. Be your own doctor.

10. **Exercise:** Not only will this aid every system in the body, it will also help the movement – the peristalsis – of food through the digestive tract. A spot of movement every day will keep you lean and efficient and in flow.

Footnotes

(1) Paul Chek, *How to Eat, Move and Be Healthy!: Your personalized 4-step guide to looking and feeling great from the inside out* (Australia, 2004)

(2) Helander, H.F., Fändriks, L., 'Surface area of the digestive tract – Revisited', *Scandinavian Journal of Gastroenterology* (London, 2014).

(3) Spector, T., *The Diet Myth* (Croydon, 2016).

(4) World Health Organization, 'Japan has the highest life expectancy – the World Health Statistics 2017 report', www.who.int/kobe_centre/mediacentre/whs/en/ (accessed on 10/01/2016).

(5) Perlmutter, D., Loberg, K., *Grain Brain* (London, 2013).

(6) Bercik, P. et al, 'Microbiota and host determinants of behavioural phenotype in maternally separated mice', *Nature Communications* (London, 2015).

(7) Knight, R. et al, 'Gut Microbes and the Brain: Paradigm Shift in Neuroscience', *The Journal of Neuroscience* (Washington, 2014).

(8) Imhann, F. et al, 'Proton pump inhibitors affect the gut microbiome', *Gut* (London, 2016).

CONCLUSION

How to be the best possible you

Nutrition is the doctor of the future: if you want to feel better, eat better food. If you want better skin, drink more filtered water. If you want to change your body shape, move your body until it sweats. And if you want to have more energy, seek to find a better quality of sleep, by getting into bed earlier – preferably without your phone!

Disease in the body is created largely by the food we eat and the lifestyle choices we make. When you take responsibility for your wellness, when you seek to educate yourself about health, when you change your lifestyle traits to improve what isn't working, and when you change your behaviour around how you think, what your needs, values and purpose are, you cease to become so dependent on a healthcare system that cures you through drugs only. This is when the journey to the best possible you begins and the endless possibilities of life present themselves.

True healthcare reform starts in the kitchen. You cannot outrun a bad diet. What I mean is, you can do all the exercise in the world but ultimately it's all about what you eat! Many people consider that it's getting harder and harder to eat well and easier and easier to eat badly, but that's not true, it is very easy to eat well. Making a poor food choice is seen as a treat, and we all deserve a treat, don't we, because we work so hard and we are all so stressed? Except that every day soon becomes a treat day as our stress levels elevate and stay elevated, so the food of choice becomes the food that has been heated, treated, injected, sprayed with pesticides and preservatives, coloured, washed in chlorine, vacuum-packed, shipped and flown thousands of miles to be hurriedly thrown in a microwave. We kid ourselves that this is food.

We get what we tolerate

Here's how to be the best possible you in five easy steps.

Sweat: Sweat your body every day. It doesn't have to be for an hour every day, it can be for just 20 minutes: a quick hike in the countryside or some exercises in the gym. In our fat (adipose tissue), toxins are stored and you do not want to be carrying around any extra toxins in your body. So take an honest look in the mirror and take some action today!

Sleep: This is the most underrated activity that you can take part in, and one that promotes all-round health. When you sleep your body regenerates, and it helps you to lose weight. So if you have weight to lose, get into bed on time – without your tablet or phone, or the TV on. Instead, try reading your favourite children's book to your partner or to yourself and let your body relax and prepare for sleep. Turn your emails off at least two hours before bed; there is nothing you can do now except rest, repair and regenerate.

Hydrate: Water feeds every cell in your body. Drink water when you think you are hungry, on waking every morning, before every main meal you have and after every bowel movement. Drink water between alcoholic drinks and always have a bottle in your bag when you are out. Your body cries out for water all day long and the substances that you're most fond of, such as coffee, sugar and alcohol, only dehydrate you and increase your need for water.

Eat: Polyphenols are found in green tea and dark chocolate that has a cocoa content of about 70 per cent, and protects against cancer as well as improving brain function. In fact, a green tea and a square of dark chocolate can be a better pick-me-up than a coffee. Antioxidants such as blueberries and kale act against the free radicals and decrease inflammation in the body, and bitter foods such as rocket, chicory and grapefruit promote optimal digestion and metabolism. Lastly, eat cruciferous vegetables like broccoli to help keep your hormones healthy and in balance.

Laugh, love and be: The three most important things to have in your life are love, laughter and stillness. Humans are designed to love, but the greatest love above all should be for yourself: look after you first, learn to love the good and the bad and the rest will follow. Have people around you who make you laugh and learn to laugh at yourself, life is much more fun this way; it creates more flow in life and is certainly less stressful. And finally, just be. Practise being still. In this increasingly fast-paced world we live in, being still is the new art form. Know that where you are at this moment in your life is exactly the right place for you to be.

To the best possible you.

FURTHER INFORMATION

SEASONAL BRITISH PRODUCE

Month	Fruit	Vegetables	Herbs	Meat	Fish
January	apples, blood oranges, clementines, lemons, oranges, pears, pomegranate, rhubarb	beetroot, Brussels sprouts, cabbage, carrots, cauliflower, celeriac, celery, chicory, horseradish, Jerusalem artichoke, kale, kohlrabi, leeks, parsnips, potatoes, shallots, swede, turnips	bay, parsley	duck, goose, lamb, pork, turkey, venison	haddock, halibut, hake, mackerel, sea bream
February	bananas, blood oranges, clementines, lemons, oranges, pomegranate, rhubarb	beetroot, Brussels sprouts, cabbage, carrots, cauliflower, celeriac, chicory, Jerusalem artichoke, kale, kohlrabi, leeks, parsnips, potatoes (maincrop), purple sprouting broccoli, salsify, shallots, spinach, swede	bay, chives, parsley	lamb, pork, guinea fowl, partridge, turkey venison	haddock, halibut, hake, mackerel, salmon
March	bananas, blood oranges, lemons, oranges, rhubarb	beetroot, cauliflower, kale, leeks, purple sprouting broccoli, salsify, wild nettles	bay, chives, parsley	lamb, pork, spring lamb	hake, mussels, salmon

April	bananas, rhubarb	asparagus, broccoli, Jersey Royal new potatoes, lettuce & salad leaves, purple sprouting broccoli, radishes, rocket, samphire, spinach, spring onions, watercress, wild nettles	basil, chives, dill, sorrel	lamb, pork	crab, plaice, prawns, salmon, sea trout
May	bananas, rhubarb	asparagus, broccoli, carrots, Jersey Royal new potatoes, lettuce & salad leaves, new potatoes, peas, radishes, rocket, samphire, spinach, spring onions, watercress, wild nettles	basil, chives, coriander, dill, mint, oregano, parsley (curly), rosemary, sage, sorrel, tarragon	lamb, pork	cod, crab, haddock, plaice, prawns, salmon, sardines, sea trout
June	apricots, blueberries, cherries, peaches, strawberries	asparagus, aubergine, beetroot, broad beans, broccoli, carrots, chillies, courgettes, fennel, French beans, garlic, Jersey Royal new potatoes, kohlrabi, lettuce & salad leaves, mangetout, new potatoes, onions, pak choi, peas, radishes, rocket, runner beans, samphire, spinach, spring onions, tomatoes, turnips, watercress, wild nettles	basil, chives, coriander, dill, elderflowers, mint, nasturtium, oregano, parsley (curly), parsley (flat-leaf), rosemary, sage, sorrel, tarragon, thyme	lamb, pork	cod, crab, haddock, halibut, plaice, pollock, prawns, salmon, sardines, sea bream, sea trout

July	apricots, blueberries, cherries, melons, peaches, strawberries	artichoke, aubergine, beetroot, broad beans, broccoli, carrots, chillies, courgettes, fennel, French beans, garlic, Jersey Royal new potatoes, kohlrabi, lettuce & salad leaves, mangetout, new potatoes, onions, pak choi, peas, radishes, rocket, runner beans, samphire, spinach, spring onions, tomatoes, turnips, watercress, wild nettles	basil, chervil, chives, coriander, dill, elderflowers, oregano, mint, nasturtium, parsley (curly), parsley (flat-leaf), rosemary, sage, sorrel, tarragon, thyme	lamb, pork	cod, crab, Dover sole, haddock, halibut, mackerel, plaice, pollock, prawns, salmon, sardines, sea bream, sea trout
August	apricots, blueberries, cherries, figs, melons, nectarines, peaches, plums, raspberries, strawberries	artichoke, aubergine, beetroot, broad beans, broccoli, carrots, chillies, courgettes, cucumber, fennel, French beans, garlic, kohlrabi, lettuce & salad leaves, mangetout, marrow, onions, pak choi, peas, peppers, potatoes (maincrop), radishes, rocket, runner beans, spring onions, sweetcorn, tomatoes, turnips, watercress, wild mushrooms	basil, chives, coriander, mint, oregano, parsley (curly), parsley (flat-leaf), rosemary, sage, sorrel, tarragon, thyme	beef, lamb, pork, venison	cod, crab, haddock, halibut, mackerel, monkfish, plaice, pollock, prawns, salmon, sardines, sea bass (wild), sea bream, sea trout

September	apples, blackberries, figs, grapes, melons, nectarines, peaches, pears, plums, raspberries	artichoke, aubergine, beetroot, broccoli, butternut squash, carrots, celeriac, celery, chillies, courgettes, cucumber, fennel, French beans, garlic, kale, kohlrabi, leeks, lettuce & salad leaves, mangetout, marrow, onions, pak choi, peppers, potatoes (maincrop), pumpkin, radishes, rocket, runner beans, shallots, spring onions, sweetcorn, tomatoes, turnips, watercress, wild mushrooms	chives, coriander, mint, oregano, parsley (curly), parsley (flat-leaf), rosemary, sage, sorrel, thyme	beef, grouse, lamb, pheasant, pork, turkey, venison	cod, crab, haddock, halibut, hake, mackerel, monkfish, plaice, pollock, prawns, sea bass (wild), sea bream
October	apples, blackberries, figs, grapes, pears	artichoke, beetroot, broccoli, butternut squash, celeriac, celery, chicory, chillies, fennel, garlic, horseradish, Jerusalem artichoke, kale, kohlrabi, leeks, lettuce & salad leaves, marrow, parsnips, potatoes (maincrop), pumpkin, radishes, rocket, runner beans, salsify, shallots, swede, sweetcorn, tomatoes, turnips, watercress, wild mushrooms	chives, parsley (curly), rosemary, sage, sorrel, thyme	beef, duck, goose, grouse, guinea fowl, lamb, pheasant, pork, turkey, venison	cod, crab, haddock, halibut, hake, mackerel, monkfish, plaice, pollock, prawns, sea bass (wild), sea bream

November	apples, clementines, cranberries, pears, pomegranate	artichoke, beetroot, butternut squash, cauliflower, celeriac, celery, chicory, Jerusalem artichoke, kale, kohlrabi, leeks, parsnips, potatoes (maincrop), pumpkin, salsify, shallots, swede, turnips, watercress, wild mushrooms	rosemary, sage	beef, duck, goose, grouse, lamb, pheasant, pork, turkey, venison	cod, crab, haddock, halibut, hake, mackerel, monkfish, plaice, pollock, sea bass (wild), sea bream
December	apples, clementines, cranberries, pears, pomegranate	beetroot, Brussels sprouts, cauliflower, celeriac, celery, chicory, Jerusalem artichoke, kale, kohlrabi, leeks, parsnips, potatoes (maincrop), salsify, shallots, swede, turnips, wild mushrooms		duck, goose, grouse, lamb, pheasant, pork, turkey, venison	cod, haddock, halibut, mackerel, monkfish, plaice, sea bass (wild), sea bream

RESOURCES FOR HEALTHY LIVING

Food delivery

- Abel & Cole https://www.abelandcole.co.uk: organic vegetable boxes
- Riverford Organics https://www.riverford.co.uk: organic vegetable boxes, recipe boxes
- Farmdrop https://www.farmdrop.com: local delivery from nearby farms (London, Bristol and Bath only currently)
- Mindful Chef https://www.mindfulchef.com: recipe boxes, gluten- and dairy-free

Bulk buying/ storecupboard

- Amazon www.amazon.co.uk
- Buy Wholefoods Online https://www.buywholefoodsonline.co.uk: bulk buying of organic products
- Goodness Direct www.goodnessdirect.co.uk: online health food store
- Steenbergs https://steenbergs.co.uk: great organic herbs and spices

Health food shops

- Planet Organic (stores across London selling a great range of fresh and store-cupboard foods; can also shop online)
- Whole Foods (various stores across the UK, mostly in London)
- Holland & Barrett (countrywide)

Farmers' markets

- London-based farmers' markets here: lfm.org.uk

Bone broth

- Ossa bone broth http://ossaorganic.com
- Borough Broth Company http://www.boroughbroth.co.uk

Fermented foods

Sauerkrauts, kimchi and fermented foods

- Eaten Alive https://www.eatenalive.co.uk
- Hurly Burly http://hurlyburlyfoods.com
- Laurie's Sauerkraut http://www.lauriesfoods.co.uk

Beauty products

The companies below are good sites to purchase natural beauty products:

- Content Beauty and Wellbeing https://www.contentbeautywellbeing. com
- Neal's Yard Remedies http://www.nealsyardremedies.com
- Green People https://www.greenpeople.co.uk
- Natracare http://www.natracare.com: organic unbleached and unscented personal hygiene products, stocked online and in stores all around the UK

Household products

- Dr Bronner's Castile soap https://www.drbronner.co.uk: can be used in many household cleaning tasks
- Attitude Living https://www.attitudeliving.com: do a great variety of household hypoallergenic products. Available on Ocado
- Ecover Zero https://www.ecoverdirect.com/departments/zero.aspx? deptid=ZERO: wide range of fragrance-free household products, great for sensitive skin

Linen

The below companies specialise in allergen-free, organic bedding, great for those with allergies and/or eczema:

The Fine Cotton Company https://www.thefinecottoncompany.com
Bamboo Bed Sheets https://bamboobedsheets.co.uk

Fou furnishings https://foufurnishings.com

Water filters

Nikken http://www.nikkenwellbeing.co.uk

PRACTITIONER RECOMMENDATIONS:

(N.B unless otherwise stated, these practitioners are UK-based)
Specialists

James Duffin: Integrative Neuromuscular Therapist: www.58south moltonstreet.co.uk

Alex Fugallo: Osteopath: http://beyond-health.co.uk

David Phoenix: Acupuncturist: www.zenmonkey.space

Tommo Littlewood (Dubai): Neuro Kinetic Therapy: https://balanced-bodymind.com

Andrew Mayers: Sports Massage Therapist: http://www.andrewmayers.co.uk

Mark Zawadski: CHEK Practitioner: www.peakconditioning.org

Doctors:

Dr Wendy Denning: http://www.thehealthdoctors.co.uk

Dr Natalie Greenwold: Specialty Doctor and Honorary Lecturer at the UCLH Preterm Birth Clinic.

Dr Omar Amin Ph.D.: Founder of PCI and Professor of Parasitology: www.parasitetesting.com

Dr Rafael Orti Rodríguez (Spain): Consultant Surgeon at the Hospital Universitario Nuestra Señora de Candelaria

Dr Jonathan Rees: Consultant Rheumatologist and Sports Physician: www.fortiusclinic.com

Dr Colin Natali: Consultant Orthopaedic and Spinal Surgeon: http://www.thelisterhospital.com/consultant-search/mr-colin-natali/

Clinics:
The Fortis Clinic: https://www.fortiusclinic.com
The C.H.E.K Institute: https://chekinstitute.com
The Waterhouse Clinic: http://www.waterhouseyoung.com
58 South Molton Street: https://58southmoltonstreet.co.uk
Acumedica: http://www.acumedic.com

Clinical Testing:
Invivo Clinical: https://www.invivoclinical.co.uk
PCI Europe: www.parasitetesting.com
Dutch Testing: https://dutchtest.com

INDEX

BIBLIOGRAPHY

Barnett, Richard, *The Sick Rose: Or; Disease and the Art of Medical Illustration* (London, 2014).

Bernstein, Richard K., *Dr Bernstein's Solution: The complete guide to achieving normal blood sugars* (New York, 1997).

Bradley, Tamdin Sither, *Principles of Tibetan Medicine What It Is, How It Works, and What It Can Do for You* (London 2000).

Braly, James and Hoggan, Ron, *Dangerous Grains: Why gluten cereal grains may be hazardous to your health* (New York, 2003).

Fry, John and Sandler, Gerald, *Common Diseases: their nature, prevalence and care* (5th ed. Lancaster UK, 1993).

Hay, Louise L., *You Can Heal your Life*, (London, 1984).

Hilderbrand, Caz, *Herbarium* (London, 2016).

Lawrence, Felicity, *Not on the Label: What really goes into the food on your plate*

(London, 2014).

Lipski, Elizabeth, *Digestive Wellness: Strengthen the immune system and prevent disease through healthy digestion* (4th ed., New York, 2011).

Mercola, Joseph and Lerner, Ben, *Generation XL: Raising Healthy, Intelligent Kids in a High-Tech, Junk-Food World* (Nashville, 2013).

Segnit, Niki, *The Flavour Thesaurus* (London, (2010).

Smith, Justin, $29 Billion Reasons to Lie About Cholesterol: Making profit by turning healthy people into patients (Leicester, 2009).

Tierra, Lesley, Healing with the Herbs of Life (Toronto, 2003).

Ward, Lock, Mrs Beeton's Everyday Cookery (London and Melbourne, 2015).

White, Linda B., and Foster, Steven, The Herbal Drugstore (New York, 2000).

Wilson, James L., Adrenal Fatigue: The 21st century stress syndrome (California, 2002).

Wolcott, William and Fahey, Trish, The Metabolic Typing Diet (New York, 2014).

ACKNOWLEDGEMENTS

There are probably too many people to thank from the bottom of my heart, but the first group are all my clients past and present who have allowed me to help them get to the best place in their health and life. I have learnt as much from you as you have from me and I thank you for giving me permission to work with you on your journey.

Thank you to a group of very close friends who have in the process of writing this book allowed me to read endless excerpts to them, who have been there for me in so many ways over the last few years that I never expected to experience from friends. You are all without a doubt the most special people in my life and with you I am the best person I can be. Jane Camilloni, Hulya Bairaktar, Lisa Carrodus, Mr Bramble, Victoria Manslove, Oliver Bailey, Johnny Barradale, Nick Allen and Claire Wrigglesworth. Thank you also to James Duffin and Claud Serjeant, whose knowledge of the human body always astounds me. Thank you all for being sounding boards for new ideas and terrible ideas and shoulders to lean on – and for putting up with my terrible texting.

To my sister and best friend Clare Richards, who is my rock. Always there with the advice and opinions which, although at times hard to listen to, I took on board.

To Paul Chek and Emma Lane, two of the greatest teachers in health we have in the twenty-first century. I remember sitting in CHEK HLC I with Emma Lane and realising that I had finally found my vocation in life. I was 26 years old.

To Sophie Hutcherson, who allowed the dream of Move Three Sixty to exist and for me to grow into the practitioner I am today because of facilitating this dream. I am eternally grateful.

To Lisa Milton and Julia Kingsford (my agent and best friend since we were 11 years old).

To Mum and Dad, who taught me some wonderful values in life. Thank you, Dad, for letting me take over your office at the bottom of the garden in Somerset, which became my second home. Thank you, Mum, for being one of the bravest people I know and for letting me tell your story.

To the one and only Jerome Burne, laptops and odd shoes – may we one day write a book together.

To Dr Natalie Greenwold and Dr Rafa Ortiz for proofreading and becoming great friends.

ABOUT THE AUTHOR

I grew up in the Somerset countryside, where a battery-operated milk van delivered milk to the door in glass bottles with different coloured tops and eggs flecked with chicken poo in their little cardboard boxes. All our food essentials were on the doorstep; there was a farm shop at the end of the village, a village shop with post office, the meat came from the butcher – 'Mike's' is still there today – and the fish from 'Bath Place' fishmongers. Everyone knew each other.

My mother taught me to cook, and I took a keen interest from a young age – I was her little assistant in the kitchen, and I would pretend I was on a cooking show, which kept me content for hours! Herbs were picked from the garden and the pantry was full of spices, flours and Mason jars full of goodness knows what. I remember one afternoon sneaking into the kitchen pantry for a spoon of icing sugar only to have reached for the cornflour instead. I came out like Puff the magic dragon blowing smoke from my mouth. The pantry was my apothecary – shelves upon shelves of potions – and as a young girl, this image stuck with me.

It was clear growing up that my sister and I were going to follow in my father's footsteps of being athletes, following him to the English Schools' Athletic Championships. From the heptathlon and the 100m hurdles at school, I moved into hockey while at university. Sport was, and still is, a huge part of my life and continues to be a daily ritual – whether it's tennis, the gym or tai-chi, it is something I could not function without. Give me a challenge or set me a goal and I'm there, it's part of my make-up.

I finally found my vocation while sat in a classroom in the C.H.E.K. Institute, started by Paul Chek, where I was learning about Holistic Lifestyle coaching. I knew then that this was my calling. I was 26. I always thought I had wanted to be an actress, but when the lead female roles didn't flood my inbox I started to rethink – what did I want, what did I love and what was the core of me? I was being taught by Emma Lane, who became one of my most guided teachers and inspirations, and I remember the whole weekend like it was yesterday. Holistic Lifestyle coaching was right for me because helping others is what I think I was made to do.

So, I opened a holistic health clinic in 2011 with a partner and ran it for five years. It was a place designed for clients and practitioners to grow, learn, educate, make mistakes, laugh and love. It was the start of my apprenticeship of being a Nutrition and Lifestyle Coach. I have discovered many things in life so far and have been through some pretty tough times, and I know the greatest, most powerful thing you can do when life throws you off your path is to remain strong, forgive, eat well, exercise a lot and not reach for the wine bottle! This is a formula that will get you out of any tricky situation life throws at you. You have one life, one incredible body and a thousand billion chances and opportunities to create what you want, so squeeze every last bit out of every opportunity that comes your way and you will always be on the right path. There are no certainties in life, that is for sure, but with every opportunity there are wonderful possibilities. Surround yourself with people who inspire you and who are always creating and moving, and you can be the best possible you.